Atlas of Surgical Endoscopy

The Atlases of Operative Surgery

Series Editor
R. Scott Jones, M.D.
Professor and Chairman
Department of Surgery
The University of Virginia
Charlottesville, Virginia

PUBLISHED AND FORTHCOMING VOLUMES

Daly & Cady/ATLAS OF SURGICAL ONCOLOGY

Donovan/ATLAS OF TRAUMA SURGERY

Lamberth & Doty/PERIPHERAL VASCULAR SURGERY

Jones/ATLAS OF LIVER AND BILIARY SURGERY

Kaiser/ATLAS OF GENERAL THORACIC SURGERY

Reber & Zinner/ATLAS OF PANCREATIC SURGERY

Thompson/ATLAS OF SURGERY OF THE STOMACH, DUODENUM AND SMALL BOWEL

Wells/ATLAS OF BREAST SURGERY

An Atlas of Operative Surgery

Atlas of Surgical Endoscopy

by

Jeffrey L. Ponsky, M.D.
Professor of Surgery
Case Western Reserve University School of Medicine
Director, Department of Surgery
The Mt. Sinai Medical Center
Cleveland, Ohio

Illustrated by Debra Shirley

Mosby
Year Book

St. Louis Baltimore Boston Chicago London Philadelphia Sydney Toronto

Mosby Year Book

Dedicated to Publishing Excellence

Sponsoring Editor: Nancy E. Chorpenning
Associate Managing Editor, Manuscript Services: Deborah Thorp
Production Project Coordinator: Karen Halm
Proofroom Manager: Barbara Kelly

Mosby-Year Book, Inc.
11830 Westline Industrial Drive
St. Louis, MO 63146

1 2 3 4 5 6 7 8 9 0 CL PCP 95 94 93 92 91

Library of Congress Cataloging-in-Publication Data

Ponsky, Jeffrey L.
Atlas of surgical endoscopy / Jeffrey L. Ponsky.
p. cm.
Includes bibliographical references and index.
ISBN 0-8151-6742-3
1. Digestive organs—Endoscopic surgery—Atlases. I. Title.
[DNLM: 1. Digestive System—surgery—atlases. 2. Endoscopy—methods—atlases. WI 17 P798a]
RD540.P65 1991
617.4'3059—dc20
DNLM/DLC
for Library of Congress

91-22619
CIP

For Esther and Howard
who demonstrated unwavering confidence and love
and for Bennett
who showed me the way.

Series Introduction

Today's practicing surgeons and surgical educators will remember well the *Handbooks of Operative Surgery,* originally published in the 1950s and 1960s. Written by respected clinical surgeons and covering multiple disciplines within the field, this series became a very popular reference source for residents, students, and young surgeons. The careful description of operative techniques, the in-depth analysis of indications for surgery, highlights of the common problems associated with diseases and treatments, and the lucid illustrations, led to their renown.

The practice of surgery has changed dramatically since the *Handbooks of Operative Surgery* were written. Many operations featured in the series are now obsolete due to the ever-increasing pace of technology and research. New approaches have developed in their place in every field. In addition to surgical techniques, devices to support intraoperative management, diagnostic imaging, and preoperative and postoperative care have all progressed rapidly.

Responding to these changes, Mosby-Year Book, Inc, has introduced a new series, the *Atlases of Operative Surgery*. It is hoped that these will be, to the new generation of young surgeons and residents, what the *Handbooks of Operative Surgery* were to prior generations. These new editions offer complete and current material on important components of general surgery with an emphasis on intraoperative management of diseases encountered by practicing general surgeons.

This *Atlas of Surgical Endoscopy* is Dr. Jeffrey L. Ponsky's contribution to this new series. Adding an atlas of endoscopic and laparoscopic surgical procedures to the series reflects the increasing importance of endoscopic techniques to the practice of general surgery in the 1990s. Endoscopic surgery has become an essential element of the discipline, especially for general surgeons concentrating on the diagnosis and treatment of diseases of the digestive system. The application of fiberoptic endoscopy for traditionally defined surgical diseases has produced marked improvements in the quality and effectiveness of patient care.

Dr. Ponsky describes with great clarity the array of endoscopic and laparoscopic procedures that should comprise the armamentarium of general surgeons, particularly those with a significant practice in digestive disease. This comprehensive reference will help residents and young surgeons learn the techniques, applications, and indications for the spectrum of gastrointestinal endoscopic and laparoscopic procedures. Also, the practitioner will find this atlas valuable as a handy review source.

Dr. Ponsky's detailed descriptions of state-of-the-art procedures, accompanied by outstanding illustrations, effectively represent the emerging importance of this vital component of contemporary general surgical practice. It is a pleasure to include Dr. Ponsky's material in this series.

R. Scott Jones, M.D.
Professor and Chairman
Department of Surgery
University of Virginia Health Sciences Center
Charlottesville, Virginia

Preface

Endoscopy is not new to surgeons. They have been involved for centuries in the development and practice of endoscopic procedures. However, surgeons were slow to embrace the techniques of fiberoptic gastrointestinal endoscopy developed in the 1960s. These procedures were developed by gastroenterologists who became skilled practitioners and teachers of the techniques. Gradually, however, gastrointestinal surgeons took note of the value of fiberoptic gastrointestinal endoscopy and became skilled in these procedures. In 1980, the American Board of Surgery mandated that endoscopic training be a part of the curriculum in general surgical training. Since that time, endoscopy has become an integral part of surgical education and practice. It is hardly conceivable that a modern gastrointestinal surgeon be fully competent unless he has the ability to perform endoscopic examination and therapy in his own patients.

In addition to learning the techniques of fiberoptic endoscopy developed in large part by the gastroenterology community, surgeons have brought their own unique perspective and abilities to the area, developing procedures such as ERCP, endoscopic gastrostomy, esophageal variceal ligation, and laparoscopic cholecystectomy.

The present atlas is designed to schematically illustrate the basic techniques of surgical gastrointestinal endoscopy for those who seek to understand and practice these methods. Although this work is presently current, it is clear that new techniques will rapidly develop as surgical skill and medical technology continue to evolve. The future of endoscopic therapy will be dramatic and exciting, and surgeons will be at the forefront.

Jeffrey L. Ponsky, M.D.

Contents

1
Esophagogastroduodenoscopy

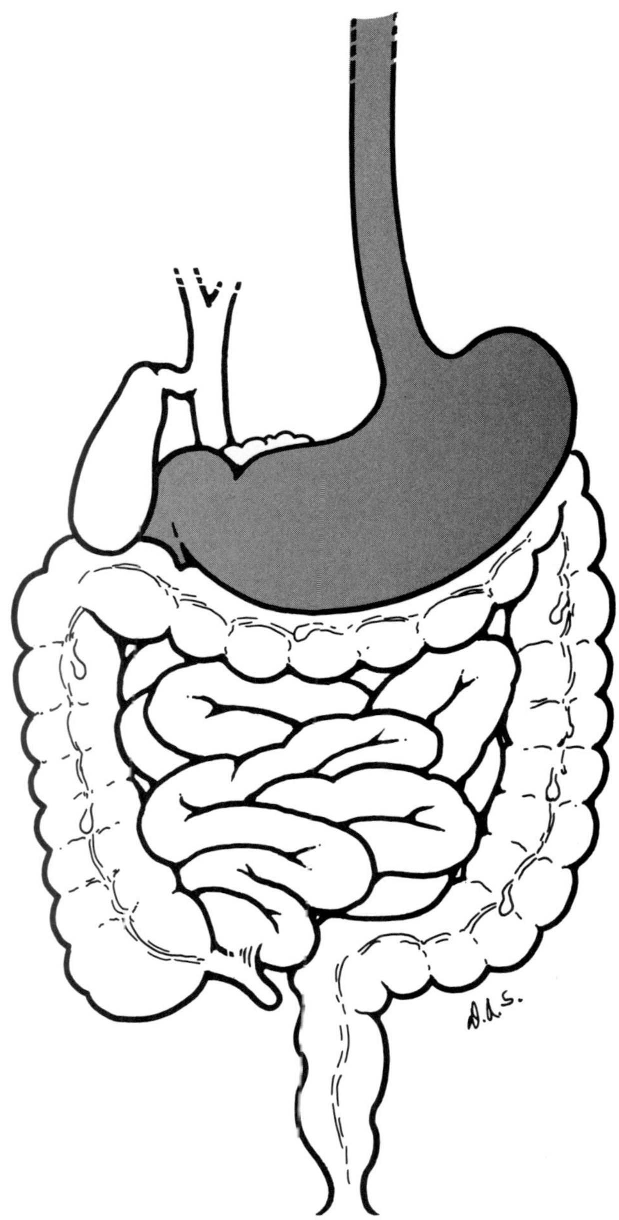

PLATE 1–1

The application of fiberoptic technology to endoscopic instruments has revolutionized the diagnosis and treatment of gastrointestinal disorders. The instrument in this figure **(A)** typifies the basic construction of modern fiberoptic endoscopes. Light from an external source is carried by means of glass fibers through the scope to the viscus being examined. The image of the interior of the viscus is then carried back to the observer's eye via a "coherent" bundle of fibers. Newer technology involves the use of a tiny camera at the distal end of the instrument that transmits a digitized image to an external television monitor for viewing. The latter obviates the need for one of the fiberoptic bundles in the instrument and yields an image of outstanding quality and brightness. Knobs at the control section of the instrument permit four-way directional control and, when used in concert, can manipulate the tip of the instrument into virtually any position. Additional controls lock the distal tip of the instrument into a particular position when desired. A biopsy channel allows the passage of accessories for biopsy and cytologic tests as well as therapeutic maneuvers. Further developments in this technology have added special lenses to the tip of the instrument for magnification, and diagnostic ultrasound has been adapted to the instrument to facilitate the elucidation of cardiac and gastrointestinal disorders.

Prior to examining a patient, the surgeon must be thoroughly familiar with the operation and capabilities of the endoscope. A knowledge of its construction and capabilities is often useful when technical problems arise during the course of a procedure. The instrument must be assiduously cleansed following the completion of a procedure. The channels must be rinsed and the insertion sheath washed with a solution of gluteraldehyde in order to assure that transmissible diseases are not carried from patient to patient. After procedures are performed on patients with known transmissible disorders, gas sterilization with ethylene oxide is effective and desirable.

The indications for endoscopic examination of the upper gastrointestinal tract—esophagogastroduodenoscopy—include dysphagia, odynophagia, persistent pyrosis, hematemesis, melena, unremitting upper abdominal pain with a normal upper gastrointestinal (GI) barium examination, and suspicious abnormalities identified on a barium upper GI series. The patient should not be fed for 6 to 8 hours prior to the procedure. The posterior pharynx is anesthetized with topical anesthetic spray or gargle. Intravenous sedation is administered slowly until the patient is comfortable but responsive.

With the patient in the left lateral decubitus position, the endoscope may be passed in one of two ways. Using one method **(B)**, a mouth guard is positioned between the patient's teeth and the scope is advanced under direct vision. The epiglottis and vocal cords are visualized and the instrument is passed posteriorly into the esophageal orifice. This technique allows visualization of the hypopharynx and may be particularly useful in patients with suspected lesions high in the esophagus or pharynx, or in relatively uncooperative patients.

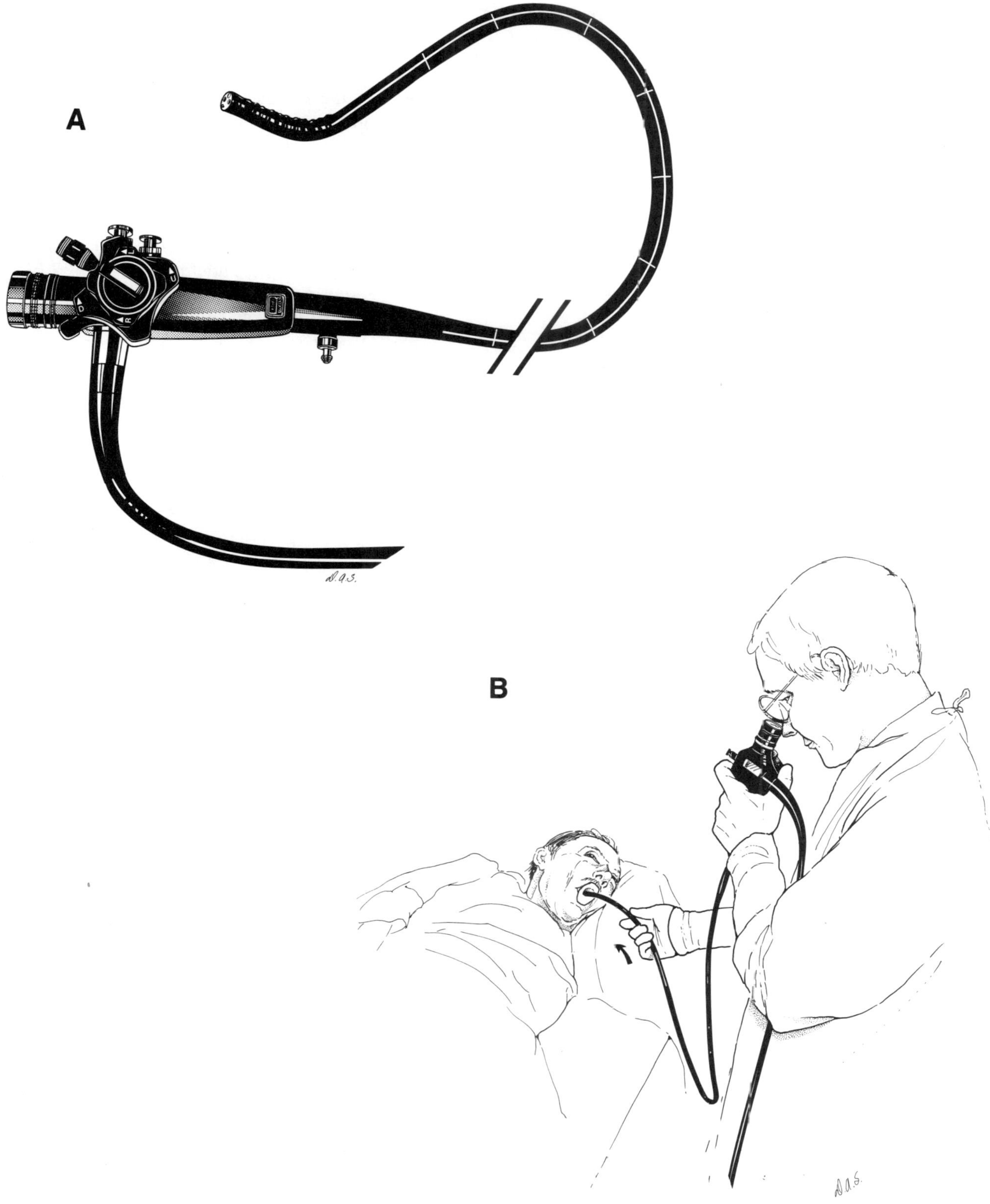
A
B

PLATE 1–2

In the alternative method **(A)**, the instrument is passed by feel of the operator. The endoscopist does not attempt to observe the lumen until the scope is in the esophagus. Observation of the upper pharynx and vocal cords awaits removal of the scope. The index and long finger of the endoscopist are placed over the tongue to the posterior pharynx. The scope is then placed on top of the fingers and manipulated downward to the esophageal orifice.

The guiding fingers assure that the scope glides along the back wall of the pharynx and is centered **(B)**. As the patient swallows, the instrument is advanced into the esophagus. Undue force is never applied, as this can result in perforation of the pharynx. The fingers are removed and replaced by the bite block. The esophagus is inflated with air and inspection is begun.

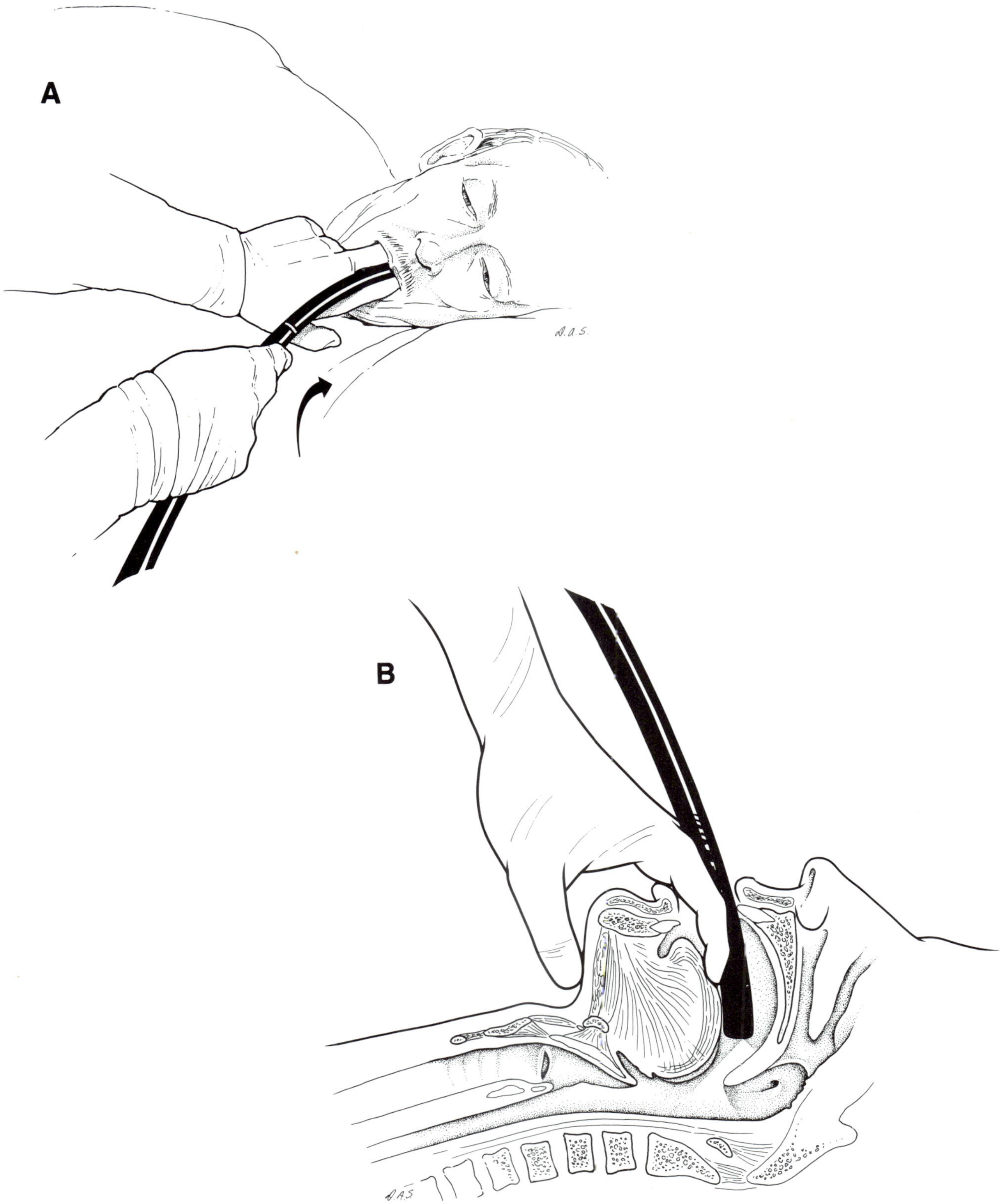
A
B

PLATE 1–3

The normal esophagus demonstrates a long, round, tubular lumen with a pale, smooth mucosa. Small, arborizing vessels may be noted in the mucosa, particularly in the distal esophagus. Careful inspection of the mucosal surfaces is important in detecting subtle irregularities that may herald underlying pathology. When any irregularity of the mucosa is encountered, it should be biopsied and brushings obtained for cytologic examination.

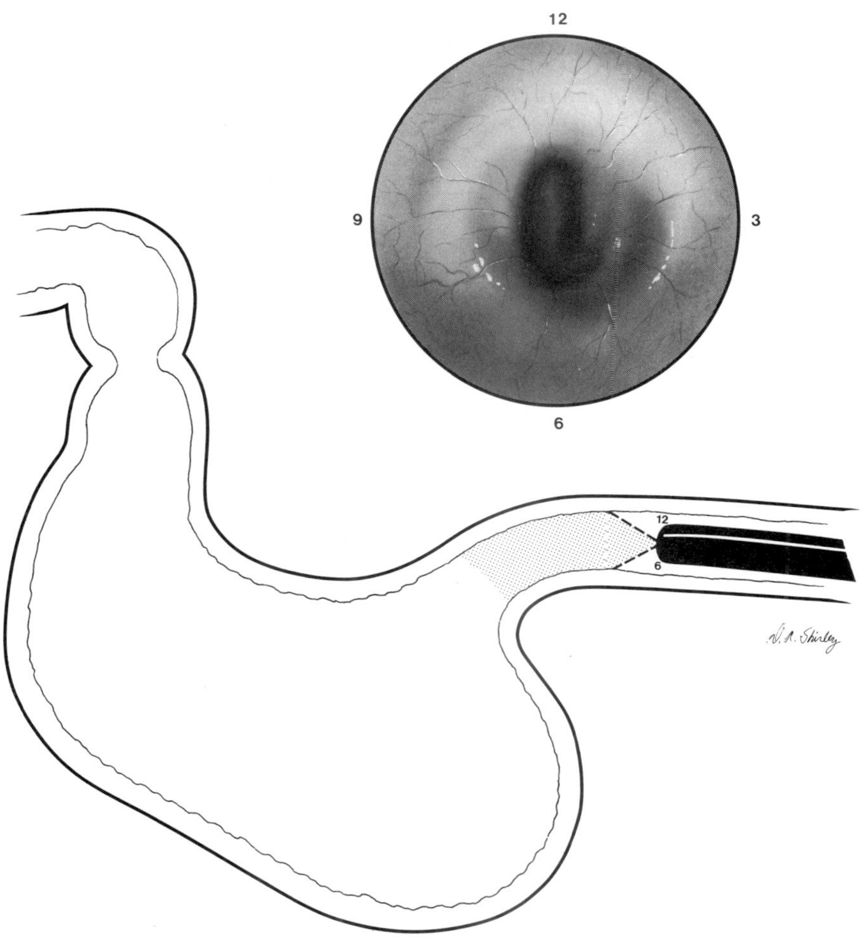
12
9
3
6
12
6

PLATE 1–4

At the most distal end of the normal esophagus, about 40 cm from the incisors, there is a sharp transition from the pale esophageal (squamous) mucosa to the deeper orange (columnar) gastric mucosa. This junction is called the *Z* line and is usually somewhat irregular. Large extensions of gastric-type mucosa above this point may represent Barrett's esophagus (columnar metaplasia of the esophagus). Such areas should be biopsied, as dysplasia and malignancy may arise within them.

The esophagus frequently veers slightly to the left as it traverses the diaphragm. The gastroscope should be advanced under direct vision into the stomach.

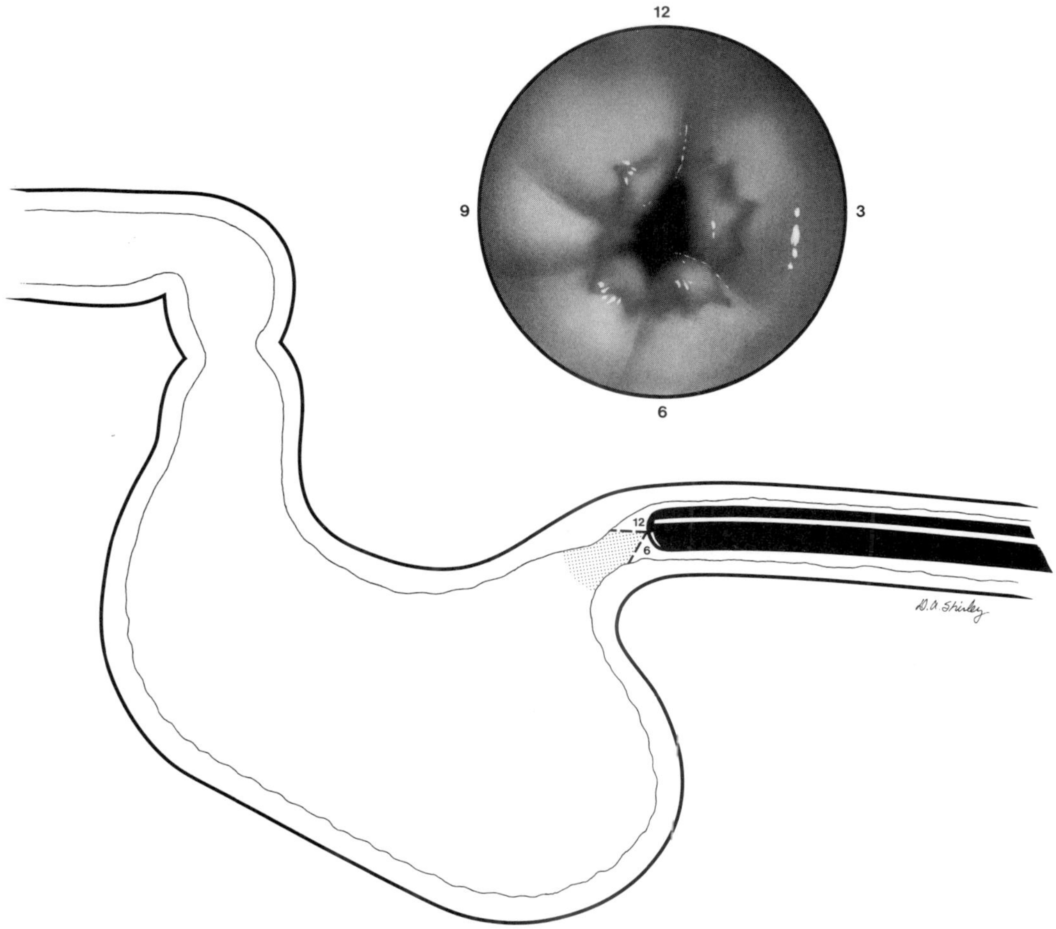
12
9
3
6
12
6
D.A. Shirley

PLATE 1–5

As the gastroscope is advanced into the stomach, the endoscopist must become oriented to gastric anatomy. The lesser curvature of the stomach occupies the 12 o'clock position in the field of observation. The mucosa in this area is usually smooth. Careful observation of the lesser curvature is warranted, as this is frequently the site of gastric ulceration or malignancy. The greater curvature occupies the 6 o'clock position. This area is characterized by prominent, parallel rugal folds, which do not totally flatten with insufflation of air. The 9 o'clock position represents the anterior wall of the stomach and the posterior wall is at the 3 o'clock position. Large pancreatic masses may indent the stomach in this area.

As the instrument is advanced further into the body of the stomach, the gastric inscisura, or angulus, becomes visible on the lesser curvature. This smooth, arching fold separates the body from the antrum of the stomach. Alteration of the smooth contour of this fold may indicate previous ulcer disease or an infiltrative process. The scope should be advanced into the antrum of the stomach after careful observation of all the parietes of the gastric corpus.

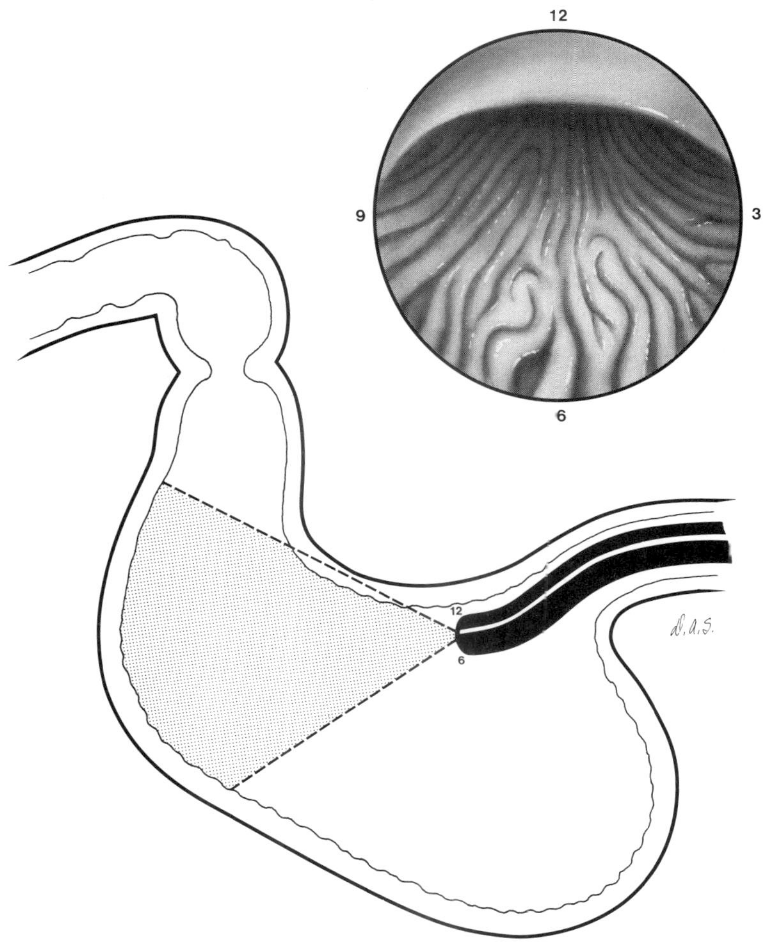
12
9
3
6
12
6
D.A.S.

PLATE 1–6

Beyond the angulus lies the antrum of the stomach. Typically, there are no rugal folds in this region. The pylorus lies at the distal extent of the antrum. It is worth waiting a moment after entering the antrum to watch the peristaltic waves pass to the pylorus. The peristaltic activity is useful in unfolding all areas of the antrum for observation and assuring that there is no infiltrative process that might limit motility. Peptic ulcerations frequently occur in the prepyloric area of the antrum.

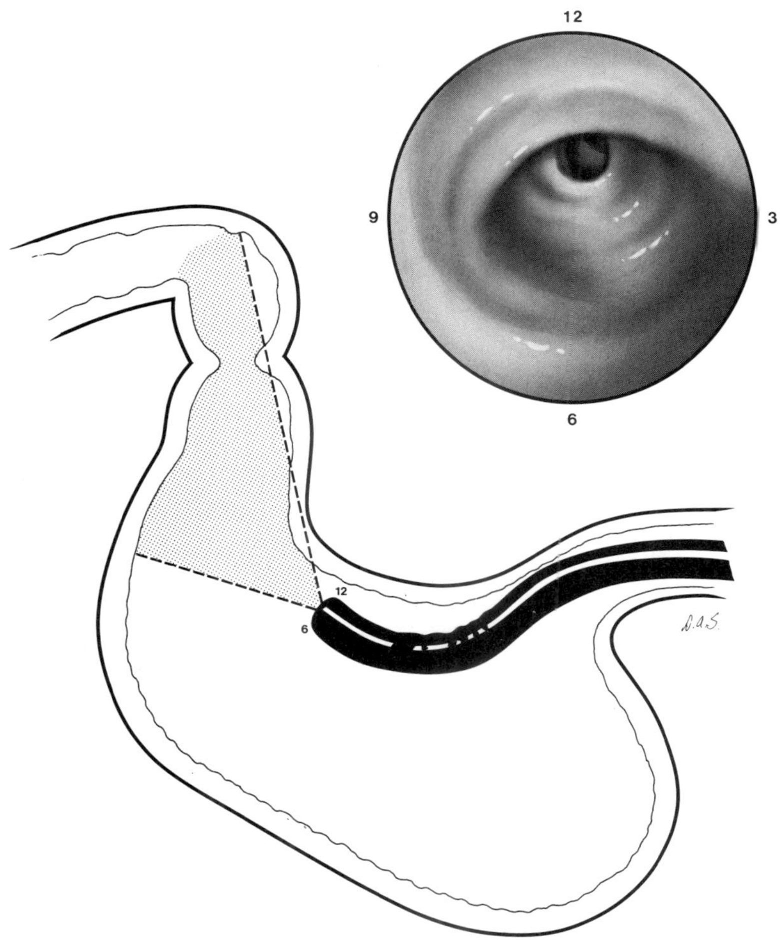
12
9
3
6
12
6

PLATE 1–7

Once positioned at the angle of the stomach, the tip of the endoscope may be turned to view the gastric cardia and fundus. This retroflexed view is useful in identifying and treating lesions of the proximal stomach. It is useful to twist the insertion tube of the instrument in this position to bring the areas surrounding the scope into view. Subtle lesions of the fundus and cardia are best identified in this manner and this maneuver must be a part of every endoscopic examination of the stomach.

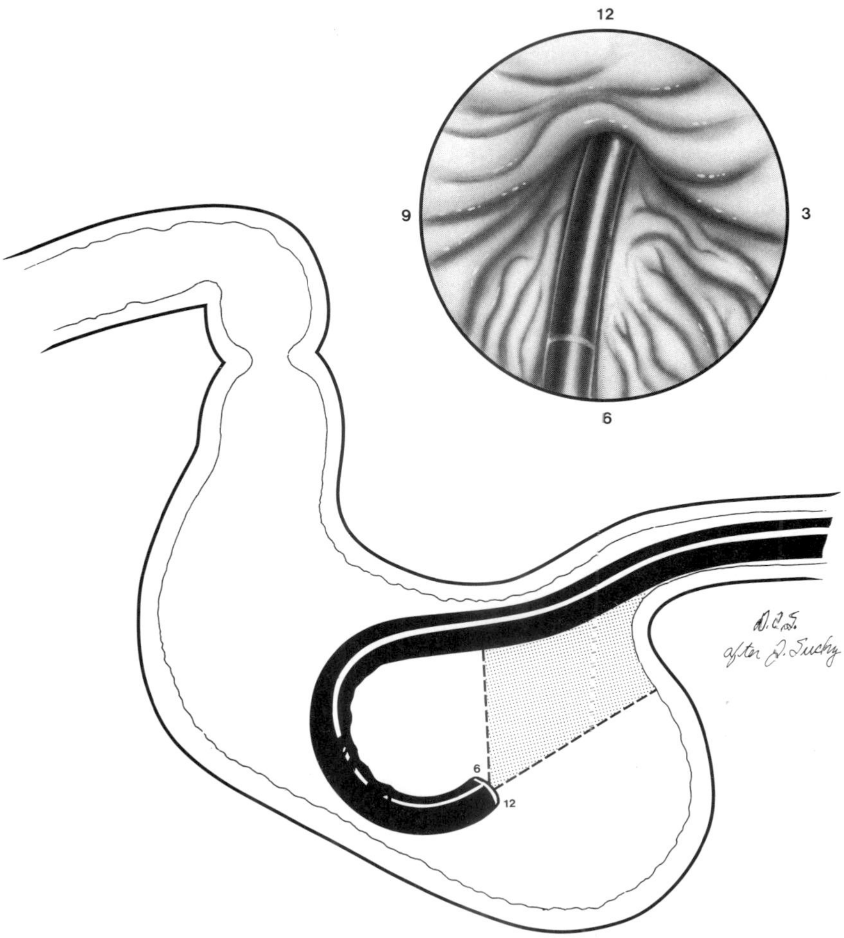
12
9
3
6
6
12

PLATE 1–8

As the scope is advanced, the characteristics of the pylorus should be carefully observed. A normal pylorus is typically round in shape and opens and closes in response to peristaltic activity. Irregularities in the shape of the pyloric aperture may suggest past or present ulcer disease. Lack of motility may indicate scarring or an infiltrative process.

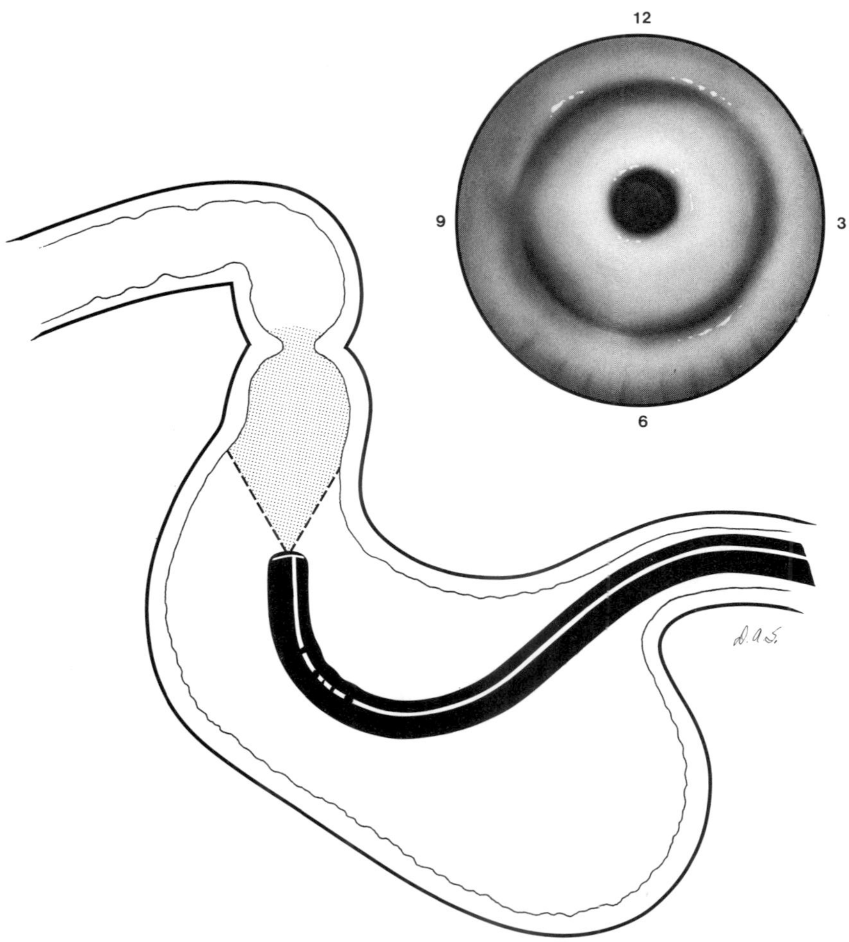
12
9
3
6
D.a.S.

PLATE 1–9

After passing the tip of the endoscope through the pylorus, the examiner should pause briefly to observe the duodenal bulb. It is not infrequent that after passing through the pylorus the scope advances beyond the bulb. The scope should be pulled back so that the first portion of the duodenum can be carefully examined.

The bulb has no folds; its mucosa is usually smooth and fine submucosal vessels are often visible. Some granularity may occasionally be present as a result of ectopic gastric mucosa. Ulcers are the most common lesion identified in this area, although other lesions such as adenomas of Brunner's gland, heterotopic pancreas, and even malignancy may occasionally be identified. The distal extent of the duodenal bulb is marked by the first duodenal fold, the superior duodenal fold. This marks the posterior turn of the duodenal lumen into its second portion.

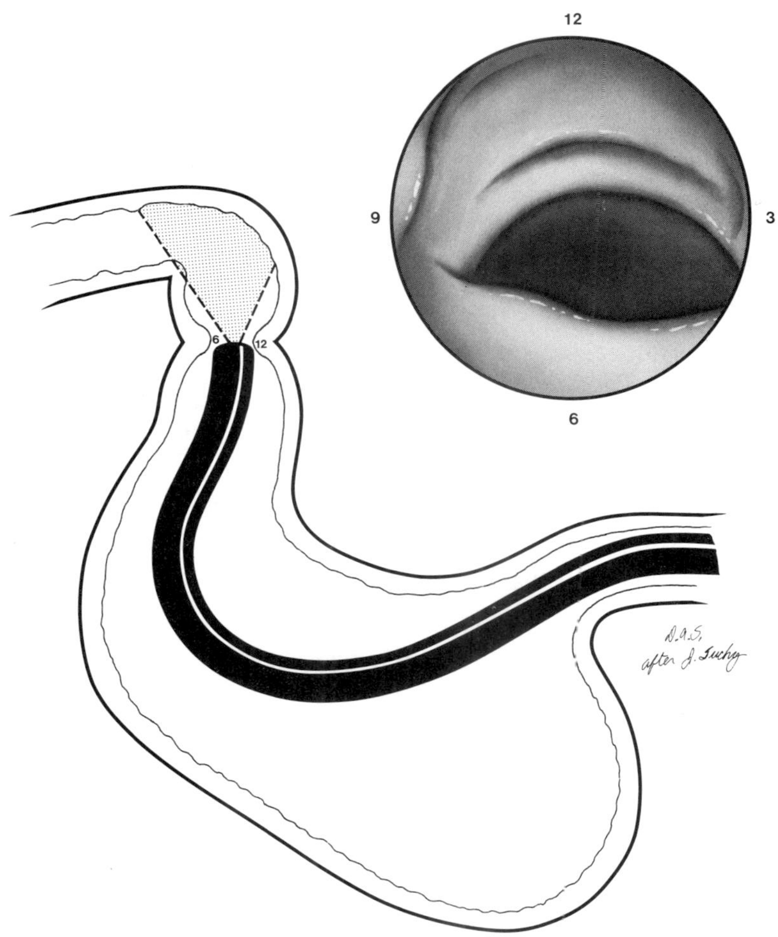
12
9
3
6
6
12

PLATE 1–10

The endoscope must be turned to the right and rotated posteriorly to advance its tip into the second portion of the duodenum. This marks the beginning of typical small bowel anatomic structure, as characterized by circular folds (valvulae conniventes). The ampulla of Vater may be noted on the medial wall of the descending duodenum; it is usually seen in profile as a small bulge in the wall.

The instrument is often best advanced beyond this point by pulling back on the insertion tube to straighten the gastric curve of the scope. This frequently causes the tip of the scope to paradoxically advance into the third portion of the duodenum. In patients with suspected lesions of the third or fourth portions of the duodenum, it is useful to employ these straightening techniques or to use specialized longer instruments to gain access to the desired area.

After satisfactory visualization of the duodenum, the scope may be withdrawn and its tip slowly rotated to examine once again the walls of the duodenum, stomach, and esophagus. Subtle lesions missed upon first examination may be identified at this time. A final look at the upper pharynx and vocal cords should be obtained prior to removal of the instrument.

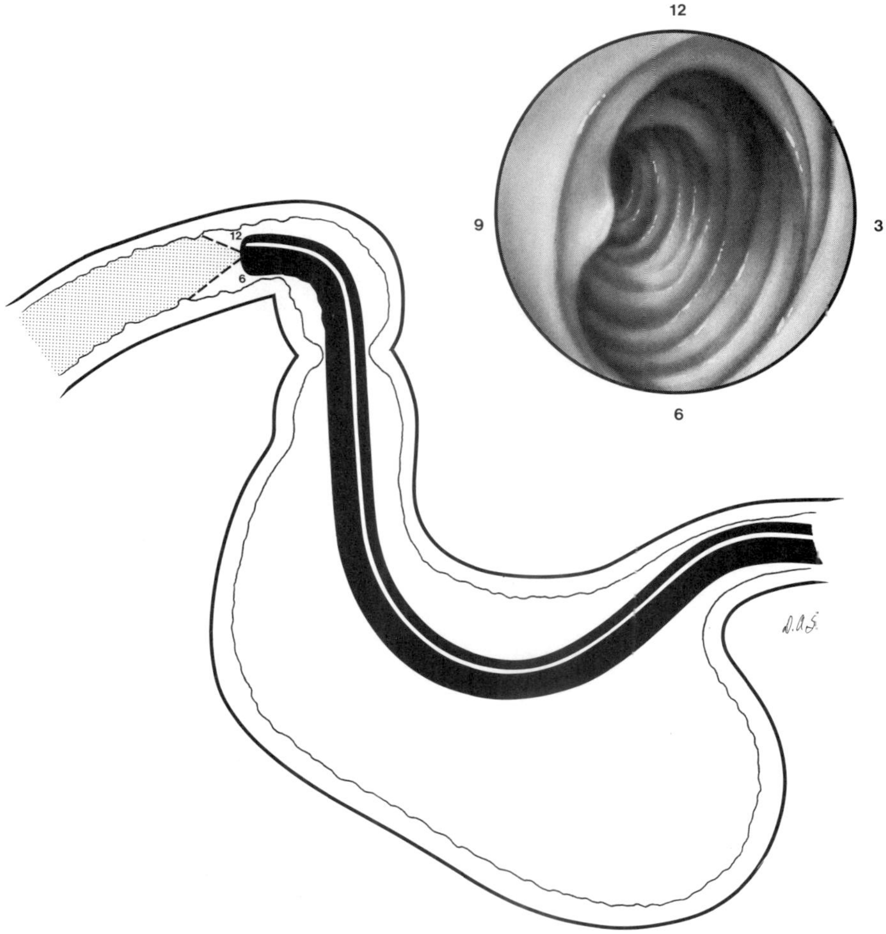
12
9
3
6
12
6

2

Balloon Dilation of Esophageal Strictures

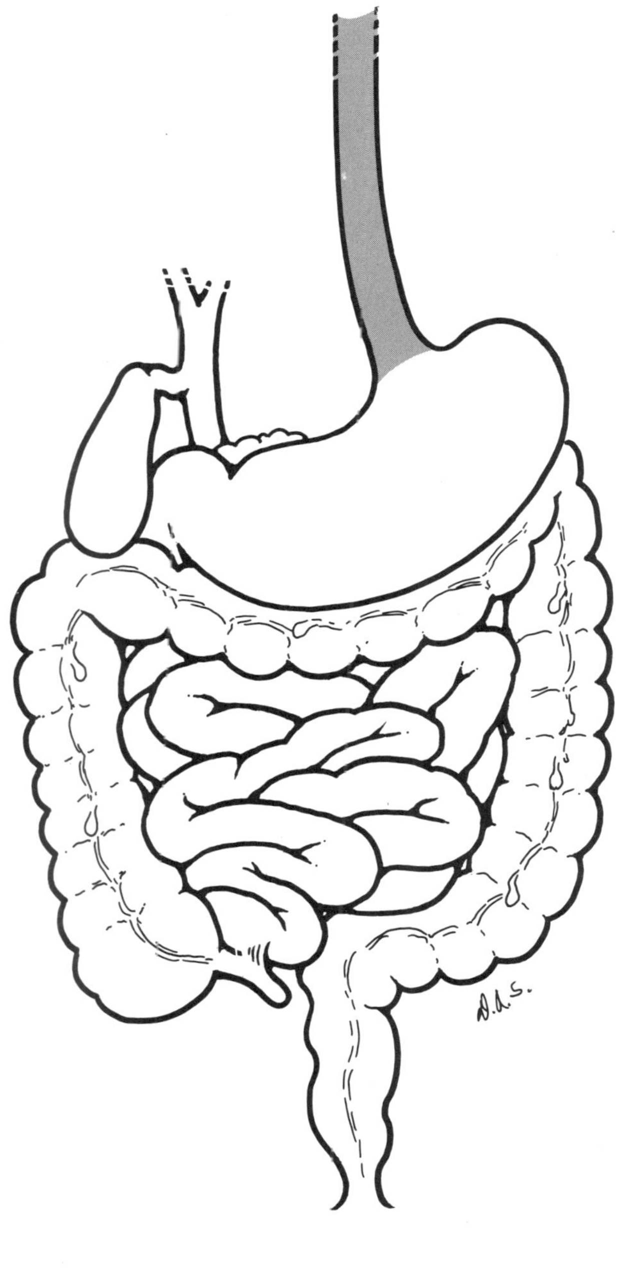

PLATE 2–1

Esophageal strictures may be inflammatory or neoplastic. At times the distinction is unclear; therefore, all strictures of the esophagus should be biopsied. Dilation of the stricture will frequently facilitate biopsy and cytologic brushings. Further, it provides treatment of obstructive dysphagia.

Strictures vary in their diameter and in their response to dilation. Some surrender easily to the passage of the scope itself or to a single balloon dilation. Others, such as those resulting from caustic ingestion, are inelastic and demonstrate great resistance to dilation. The endoscopist should assess the most likely etiology for the stricture and proceed with caution in the progressive expansion of the lumen. Excessive force must be avoided; complaints of pain by the patient should prompt termination of the procedure and a contrast study to rule out esophageal perforation.

The stricture illustrated in this plate is a common one: a Schatzki's ring (a fixed mucosal stricture), in this case occurring immediately proximal to a sliding hiatus hernia. Typically, such strictures are easily dilated. The gastroscope is positioned immediately above the narrowing and the characteristics of the stricture are noted. Biopsy and cytologic specimens of the edges of the stricture may be obtained at this time and again after dilation.

Not infrequently, strictures of the esophagus may first be recognized when the esophagus is obstructed by a bolus of food. Urgent endoscopy must be undertaken to remove the bolus, usually with a snare or grasping forceps; however, the endoscopist must not ignore the stricture that has caused the event. It may be dealt with shortly after removal of the food bolus.

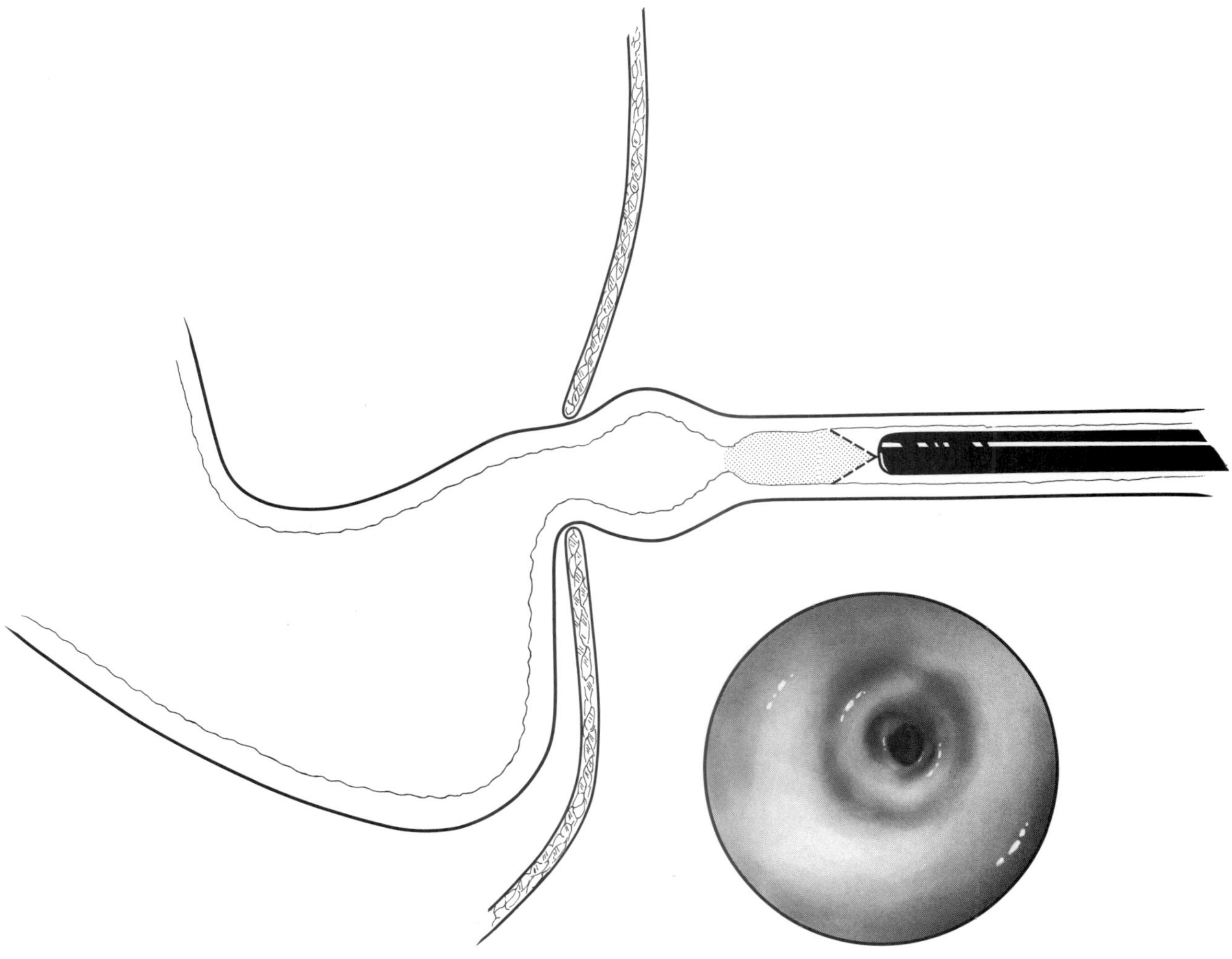

PLATE 2–2

The endoscope is positioned above the stricture; the endoscopist chooses a dilating balloon with a diameter that matches the diameter to which the endoscopist is interested in stretching the stricture in one step. The flaccid balloon is passed through the biopsy channel of the scope and positioned within the stricture **(A)**. The balloon used should be sufficiently long to span the entire length of the narrowing.

After positioning, the balloon is inflated with radiopaque contrast material while being observed under fluoroscopic monitoring **(B)**. Though this step may be accomplished using saline to fill the balloon and without fluoroscopic guidance, there can be no assurance that the maximum diameter of the balloon has been achieved without fluoroscopy.

With fluorscopic guidance and the use of a manometer on the dilating balloon to assure that maximal pressures are not exceeded (this causes rupture of the balloon), the balloon is inflated with contrast agent until its waist (the central portion within the stricture) is obliterated **(C)**. The inflated balloon may be held in this position for a minute or so to assure that the surrounding tissue has fully yielded. After the balloon is deflated and removed, the scope may be passed through the stricture, or a larger dilator used. Once the scope has passed through the narrowing, it is important to obtain tissue samples from the stricture's lower extent.

Dilation of esophageal strictures by this or any method will provide extremely gratifying clinical results; however, strictures tend to recur and further dilation is often necessary.

A

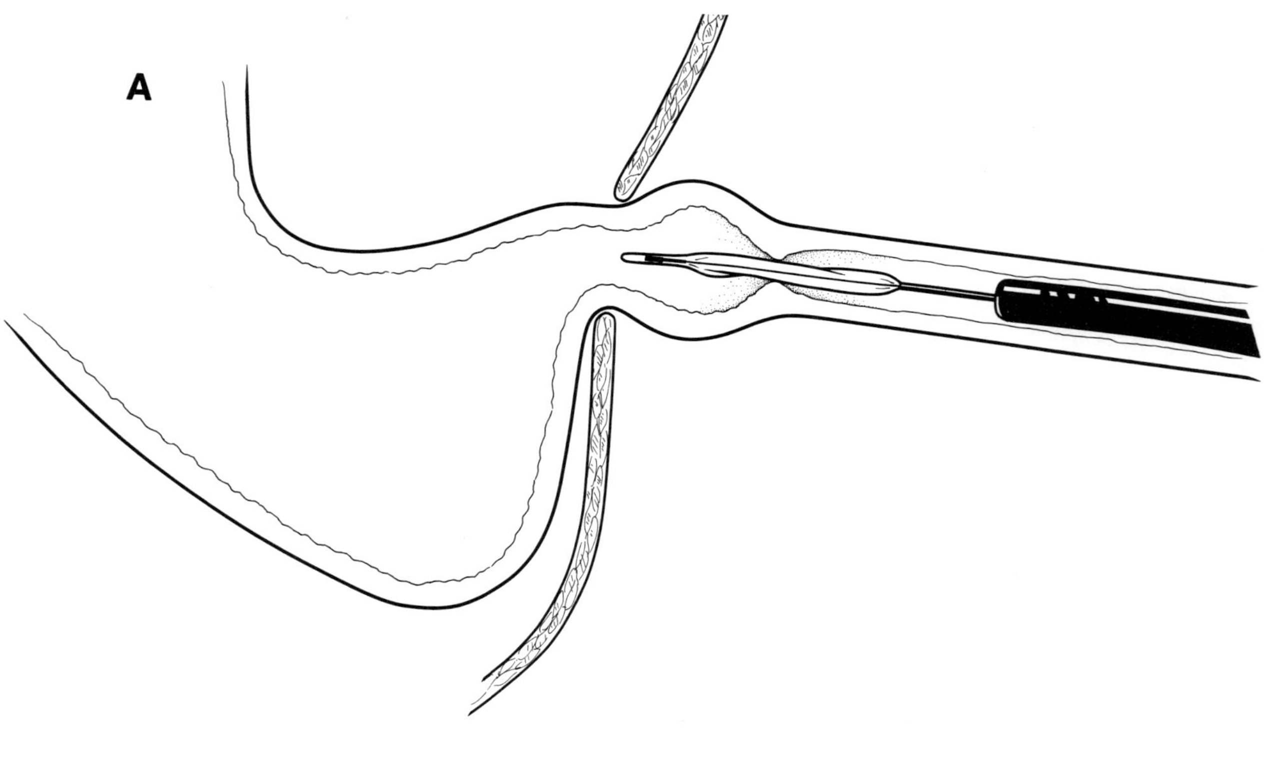

B

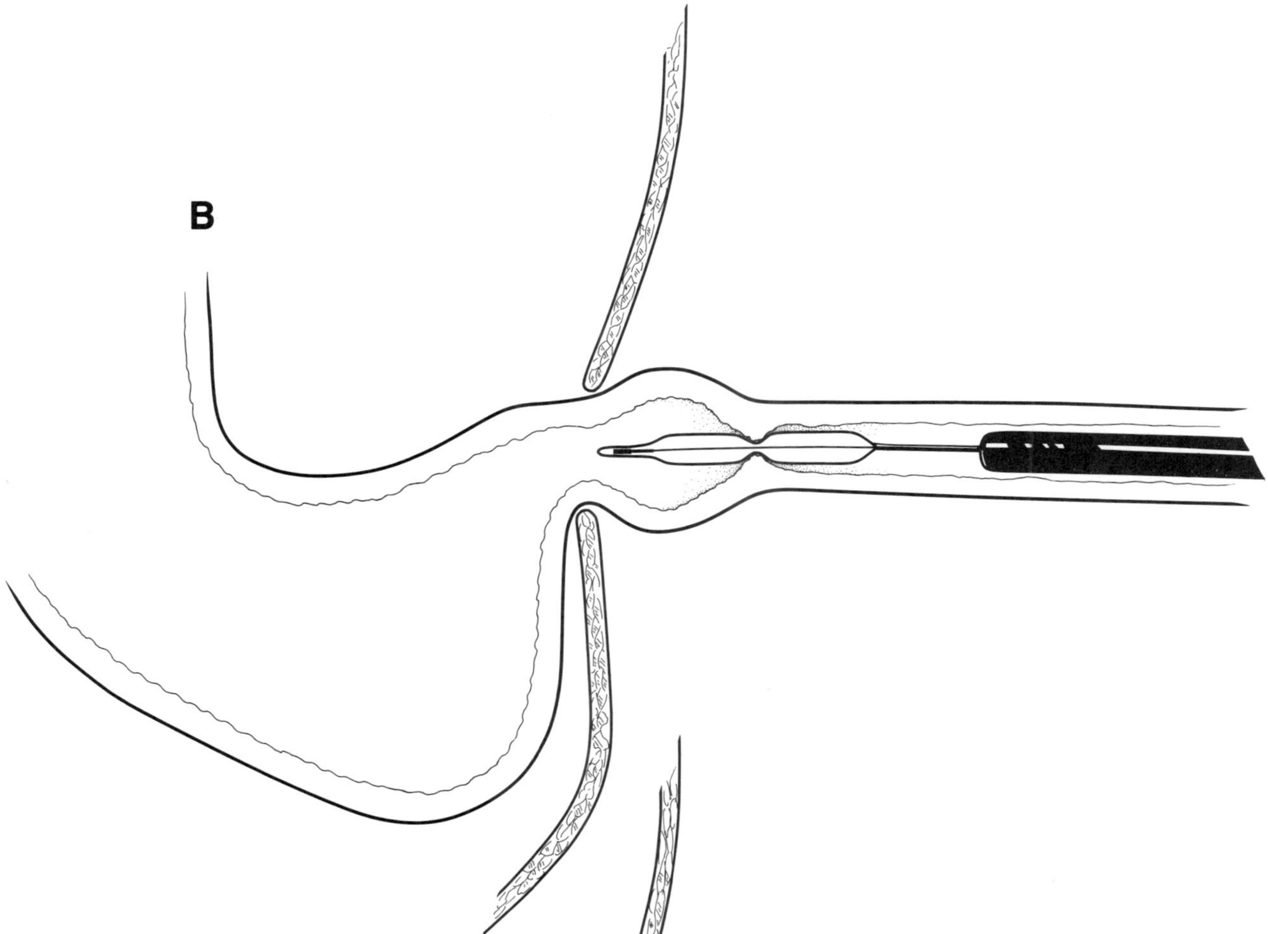

C

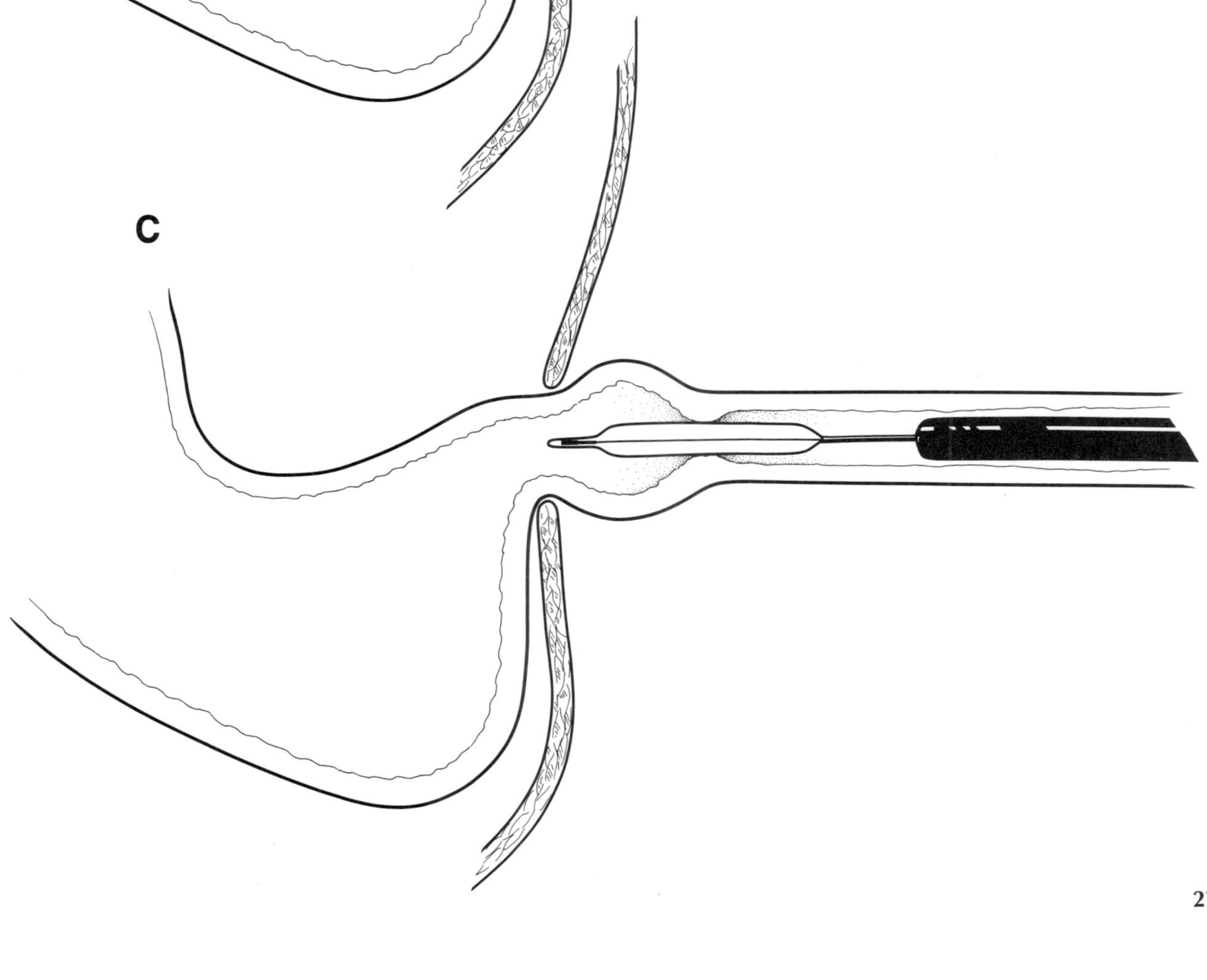

3

Endoscopic Variceal Sclerotherapy and Ligation

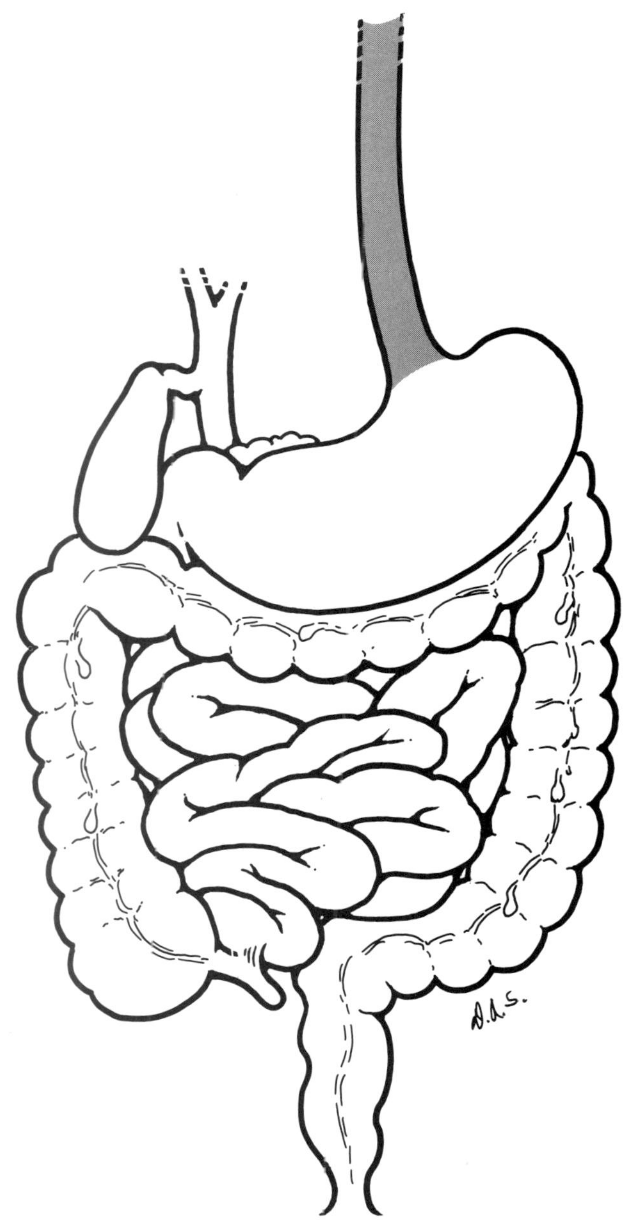

PLATE 3–1

Esophageal varices are a frequent cause of upper gastrointestinal hemorrhage in patients with portal hypertension. Endoscopically, varices appear as long columns of beadlike veins lying beneath an intact esophageal mucosal. Three such columns are usually noted. The varices are most prominent in the lower esophagus. The dilated veins represent collateral channels carrying portal blood to the systemic circulation. Bleeding from varices is usually brisk and may be life threatening. In many cases, however, the bleeding is self-limited and may have ceased prior to the endoscopic examination. Prior to implication of the varices as the etiology of a bleeding episode, other possible lesions, such as ulcer or gastritis, should be sought. Apparent gastritis in the face of portal hypertension may represent portal hypertensive gastropathy.

Resuscitation and stabilization of the patient is the first priority in treating a patient with upper gastrointestinal hemorrhage. If varices are suspected in a patient with hepatic disease, pharmacotherapy with vasopressin may be instituted prior to performing endoscopic examination.

On some occasions endoscopy may reveal active bleeding from a varix, leaving no doubt as to the site for therapeutic intervention; at other times, only a small red spot or clot on the surface of the varix may hint at its culpability. Once it has been determined that the varices are indeed responsible for the bleeding episode, the endoscopist may proceed with preparation of injection sclerotherapy. In the actively bleeding patient, only the varix that is bleeding should be treated in the initial session. Remaining varices can be addressed at additional sessions spaced approximately 1 week apart.

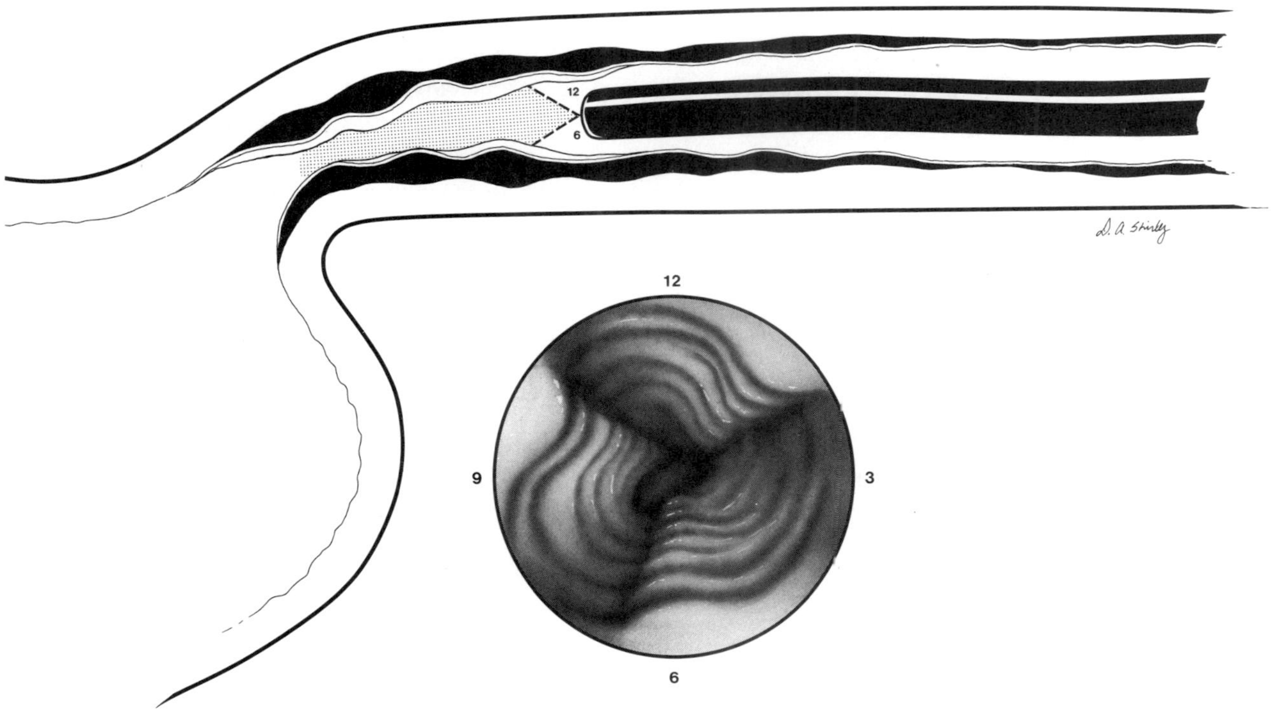
12
6
12
9
3
6

PLATE 3–2

An injection catheter with retractable needle is passed through the biopsy channel of the endoscope. The varix to be injected is identified and positioned at the tip of the endoscope. The needle is then advanced out of its protective sheath and introduced into the varix. An intravariceal injection is the goal of the therapy, although paravariceal injection may also be effective. Once the varix has been punctured, 1 to 2 mL of sclerosant solution is injected. The varix may swell and blanch as the injection proceeds. Various sclerosant solutions may be utilized, including sodium tetradecyl sulfate, ethanolamine oleate, and sodium morrhuate. In nonacute cases, all of the visible variceal columns may be injected. Therapy is commenced at the esophagogastric junction and continued proximally. Repeated sessions are scheduled as previously outlined. Examination of the injection sites at one week will reveal ulceration; this will become fibrotic with elimination of the varices. Bleeding may recur at a later date, requiring further intervention. Occasionally, in time, a stricture may develop in the area of treatment. These are most often easily dilated.

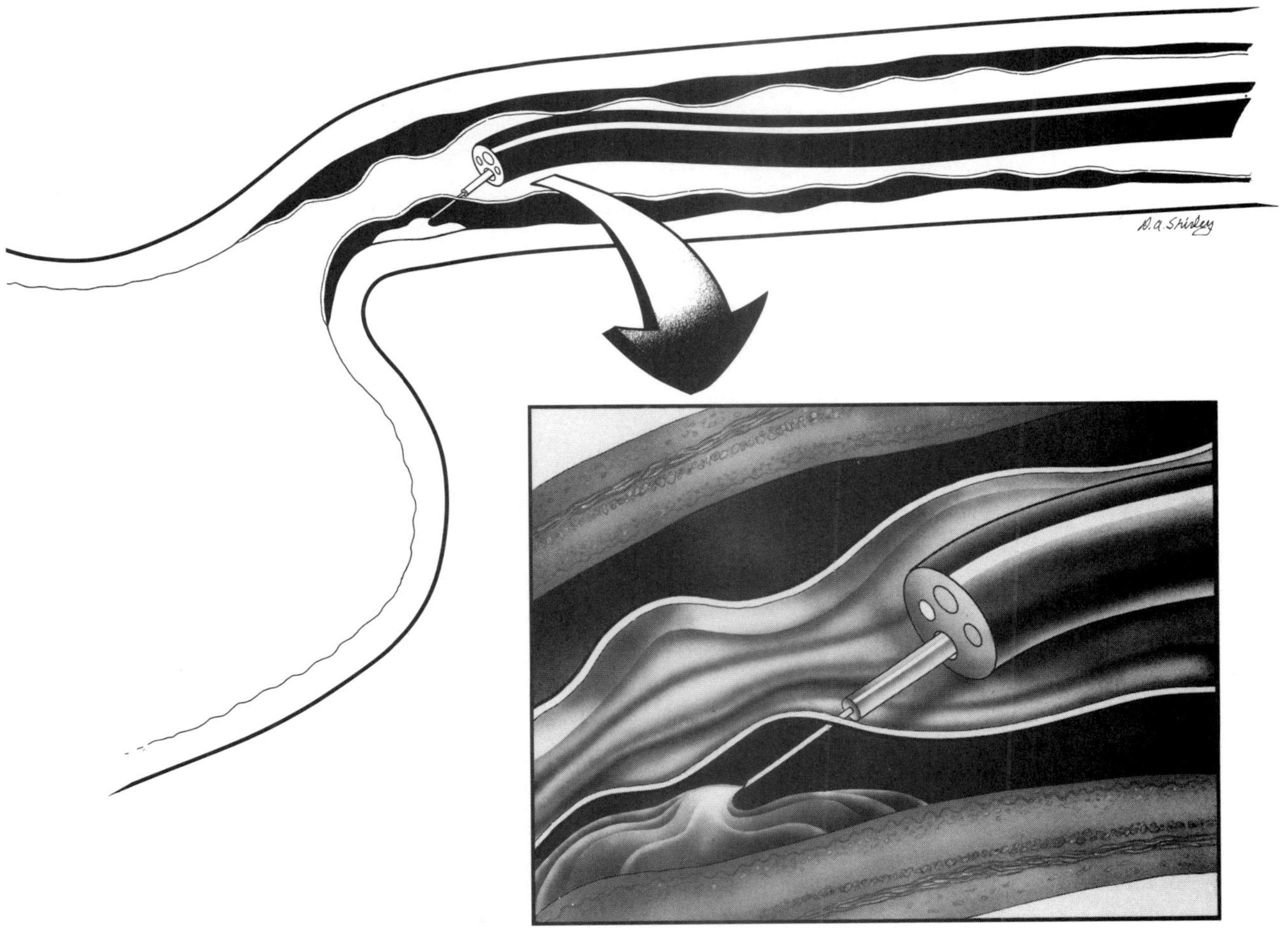

PLATE 3–3

In an alternative technique, esophageal varices may be ligated with rubber bands using a method similar to that of hemorrhoidal ligation. The ligating device is attached to the tip of a standard forward-viewing endoscope. The varix is identified and suction is applied, pulling the varix into the cup of the ligating device **(A).**

Once the varix is suctioned into the cup of the ligator, the trigger is pulled and the rubber band released to surround the base of the varix **(B).** In several days the varix will slough and its base become fibrotic. Multiple applications of rubber bands are carried out until all varices are treated. To date, results of such therapy are promising and comparable to those of injection therapy.

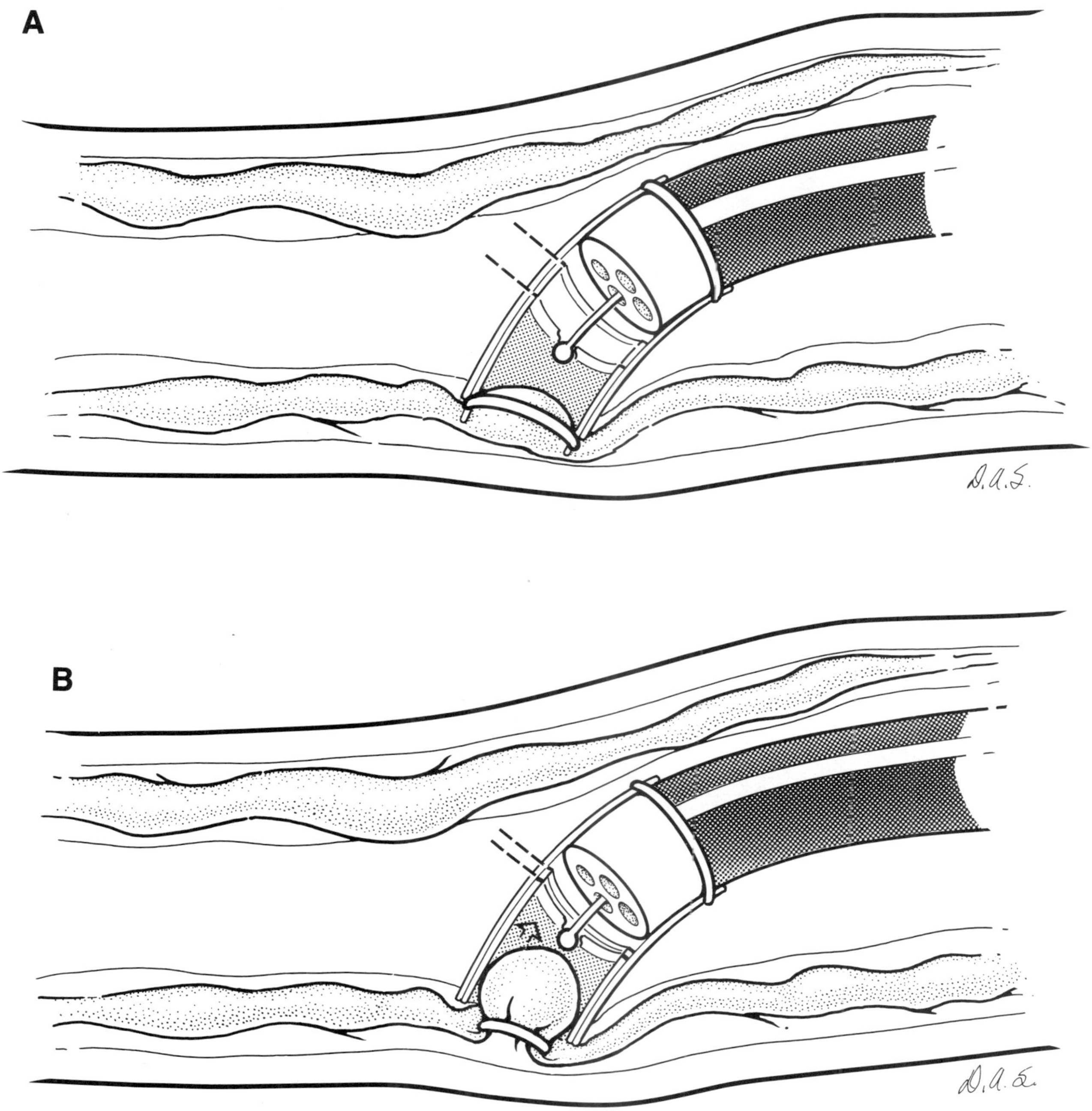
A
B

4

Laser Therapy of Esophageal Carcinoma

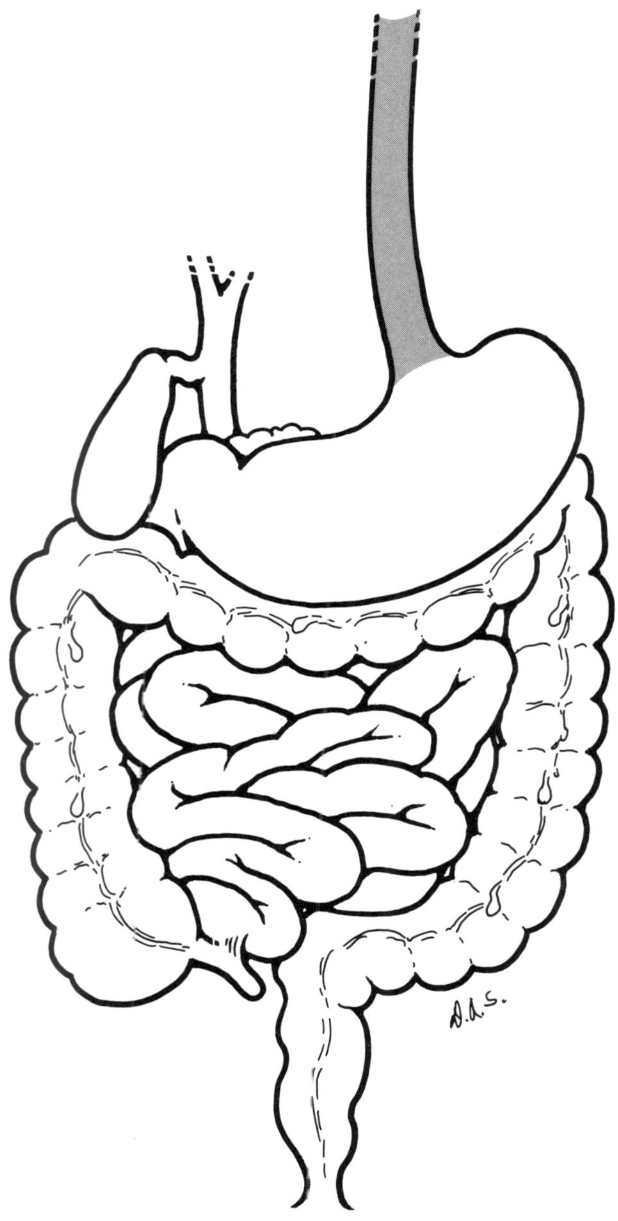

PLATE 4–1

Carcinoma of the esophagus provides a challenging treatment dilemma for the surgeon. There is certainly no question that, when feasible, resection for cure is desirable. Unfortunately, these lesions frequently extend beyond the confines of the esophagus and in most cases resection may not influence the expected survival. In many such cases it is desirable to seek palliation in the least traumatic fashion possible. The goals of therapy are the ability to maintain oral intake and control of pain. Radiotherapy and chemotherapy have been of limited value, but may offer occasional help. The surgeon is faced with the problem of maintaining a conduit for oral nutrition. Laser therapy of the tumor is an effective option. It must be understood at the outset that such therapy is palliative, not curative, and directed at permitting the patient to eat.

Prior to any attempt to treat the esophageal tumor, its extent must be carefully assessed by the endoscopist. Biopsies and cytologic brushings should be taken. When the endoscope can be passed beyond the tumor, the upper and lower extent of the lesion should be documented. The stomach and duodenum beyond the tumor should be carefully examined to identify any coexisting disease. When the tumor is so extensive as to obstruct the passage of the endoscope, the lumen position and size should be carefully noted. A guide wire may be passed through the biopsy channel of the scope and into the lumen to serve as a guide for dilation or therapy.

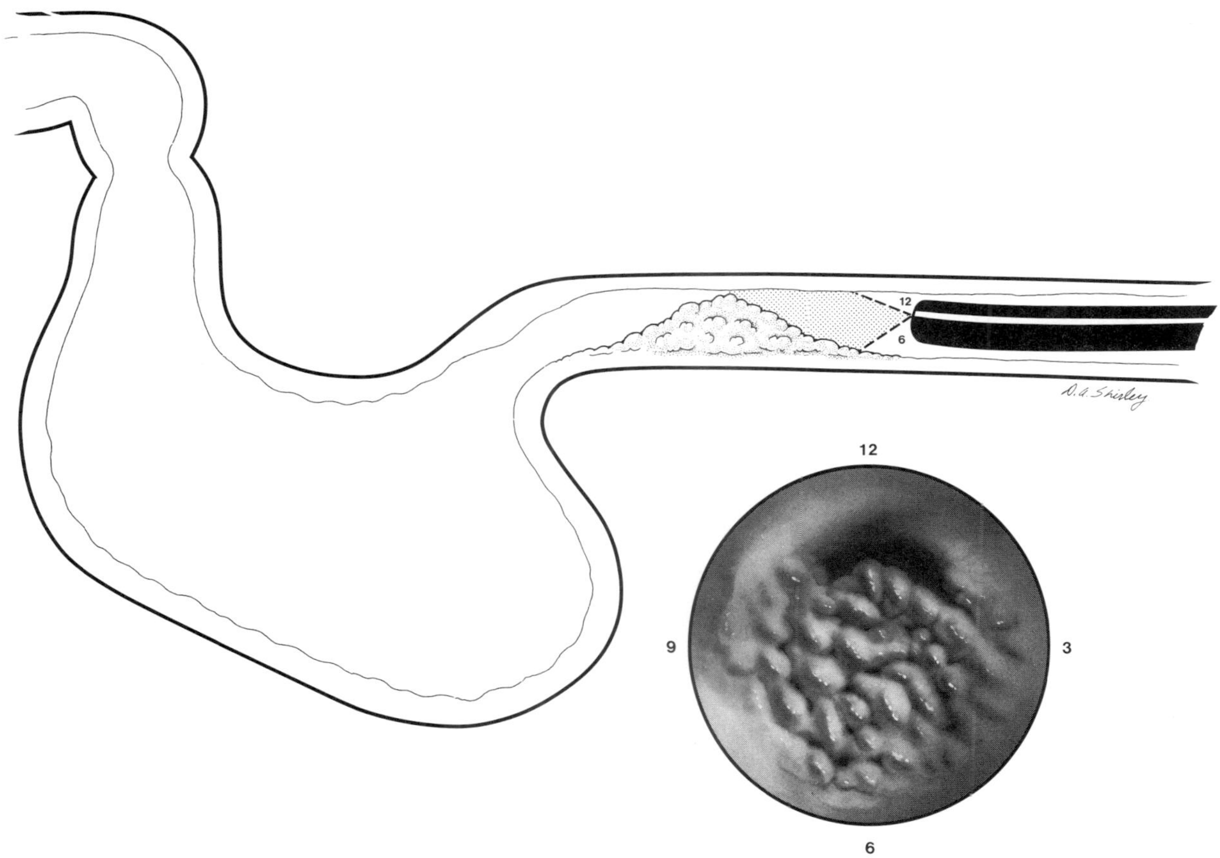
12
6
12
9
3
6

PLATE 4–2

In cases in which tumor size precludes passage of the endoscope, a deflated balloon dilator may be passed through the biopsy channel of the instrument and advanced through the narrow lumen and beyond the tumor **(A).**

The balloon is pulled back and slowly inflated in order to compress the neoplastic tissue beneath it. This process should proceed slowly, and fluoroscopic observation is useful **(B).**

The dilating balloon is fully inflated under fluoroscopic guidance. Opaque contrast material is used to inflate the balloon. Manometric monitoring of the pressure within the balloon prevents balloon rupture or undue application of force. When the waist or narrow middle segment of the balloon is no longer visible, dilation is maximal **(C).** The balloon is then deflated and removed.

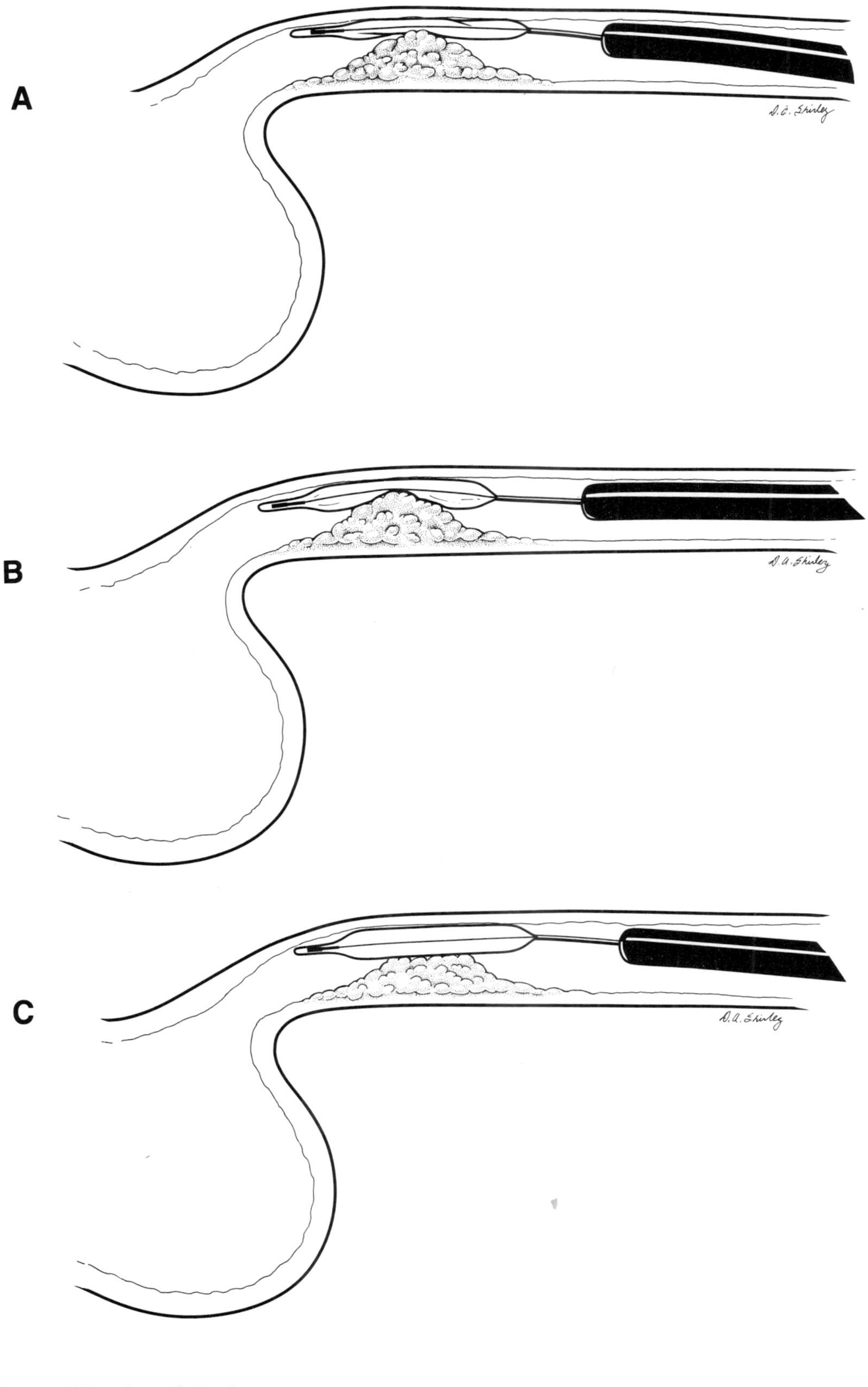
A
B
C

PLATE 4–3

Once the lumen through the tumor has been dilated, the endoscope may be carefully advanced beyond the tumor **(A).** The lower extent of the tumor is carefully noted and the stomach and duodenum examined. With the scope position beyond the distal extent of the tumor, the Nd-YAG (neodymium: yttrium-aluminum-garnet) laser fiber is passed through the biopsy channel. Various methods for laser ablation of tumor are available, including a variety of contact tips that can be used to scrape the tumor away. Most endoscopists prefer using a standard laser fiber in the noncontact fashion. Large, exophytic portions of tumor may be rapidly debulked prior to laser therapy by using a polypectomy snare and cautery.

A jet of carbon dioxide gas continuously flows through the laser fiber and may produce gastric distention. Frequent aspiration of excess gas from the stomach helps to prevent injury to the patient and to remove accumulated smoke.

With the gastroscope and the laser fiber positioned at the lower extent of the tumor, laser radiation is applied, in a "painting" fashion, to the tumor. Beginning at the distal end of the lesion permits necrotic tumor to fall or be pushed into the stomach. In this manner the procedure commences distally and proceeds proximally and therapy can be accomplished in a single session **(B).**

As the laser fiber approaches the proximal extent of the tumor, a lumen, satisfactory for passage of oral nutrients, should have been created. The endoscopist should avoid the temptation to ablate all the tumor in the wall, owing to the risk of perforating the esophagus or creating a tracheoesophageal fistula **(C).** It must be remembered that additional tissue will slough in the days that follow the procedure. It is frequently necessary to repeat the procedure at intervals when the patient experiences obstructive symptoms.

In those cases in which the endoscope initially cannot be passed beyond the tumor, therapy must begin at the proximal border of the tumor and proceed distally. In these cases the lumen must be carefully observed at all times, as perforation may occur more easily. Also, treating from proximal to distal usually requires multiple sessions to complete the therapy, owing to accumulation of necrotic debris below the therapy site.

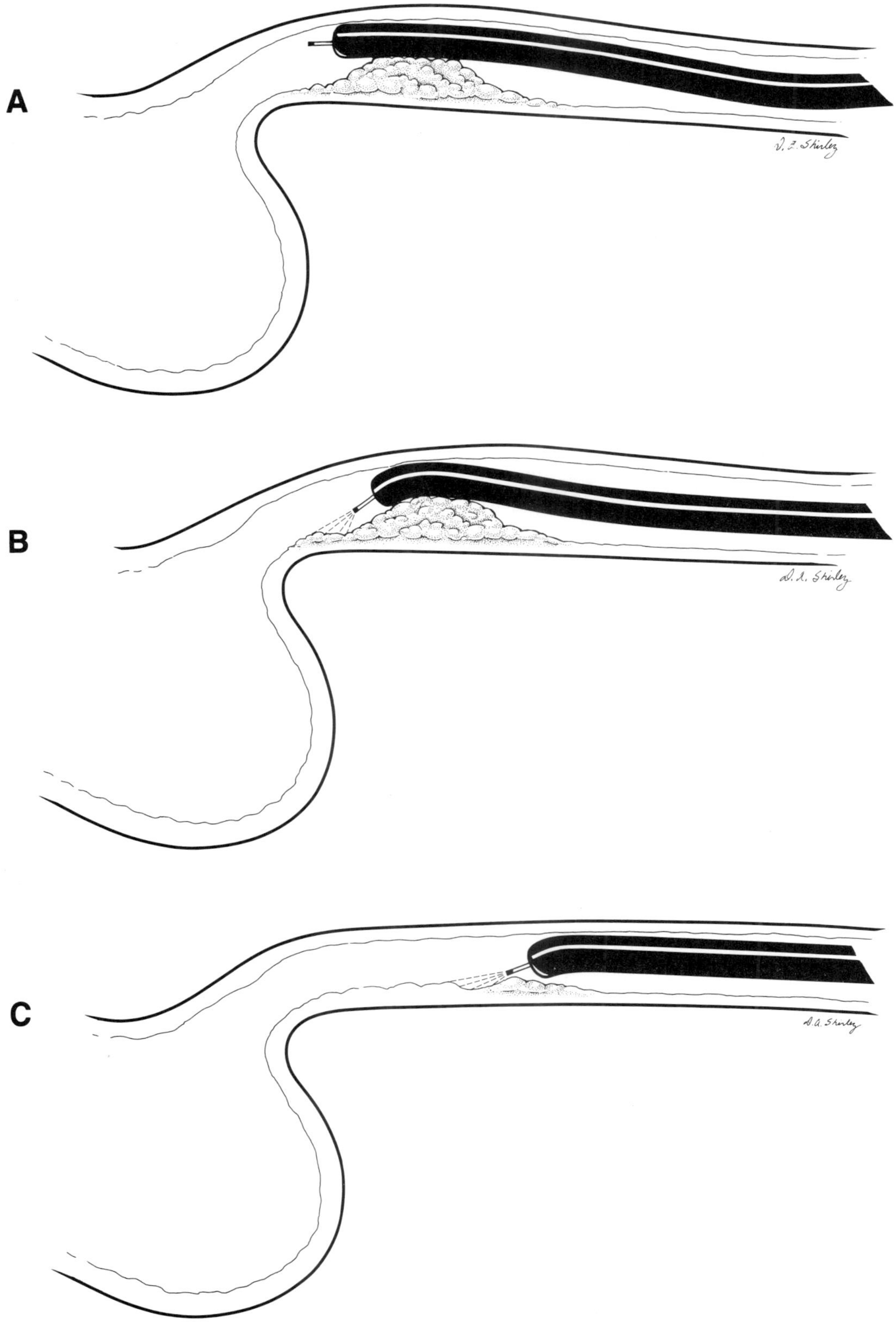
A
B
C

5

Endoscopic Placement of Esophageal Stents

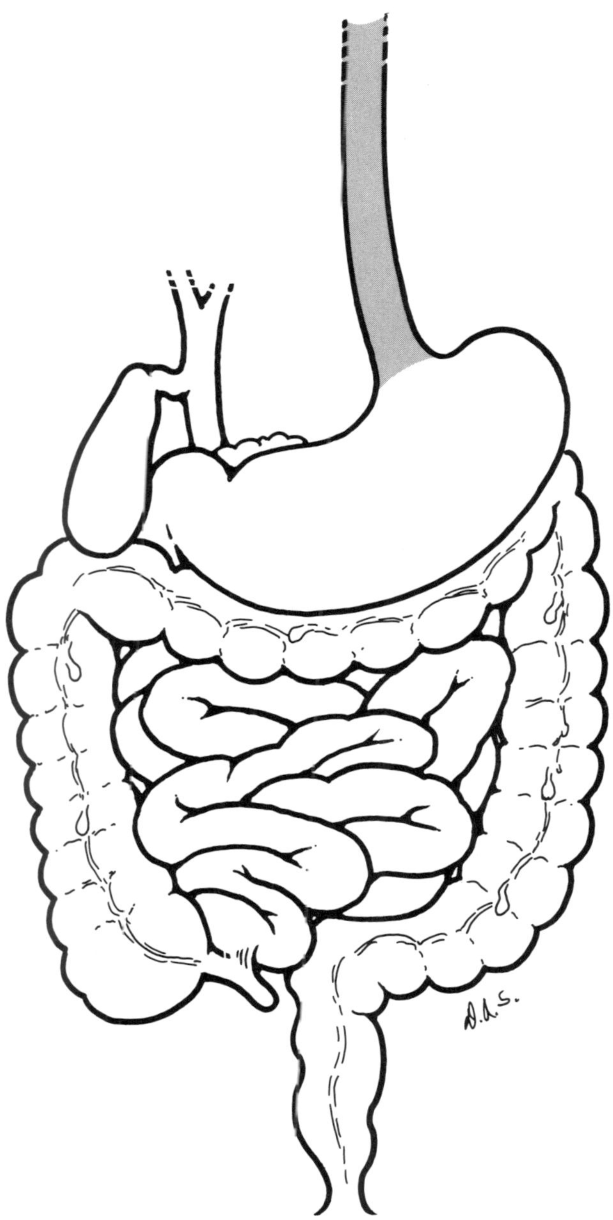

PLATE 5–1

Some esophageal or high gastric malignancies may be difficult to reduce in size by laser therapy. The necessity for frequent repeated laser treatment or the development of an esophagobronchial (or esophagotracheal) fistula may be an indication for the placement of a palliative esophageal stent. Although such stents were traditionally placed by surgical intervention, satisfactory esophageal conduits may now be established without surgery, using the endoscope as a guide. The gastroscope is first introduced into the esophagus and the extent of the tumor assessed. The upper and lower limits of the lesion should be carefully defined using the centimeter markings on the insertion tube of the gastroscope. Some dilation or laser reduction therapy of the lesion may be required in order to facilitate passage of the endoscope and the stent that is to follow; however, it is useful to allow a shoulder of the lesion to remain at the upper extent of the lesion in order to adequately seat the prosthesis.

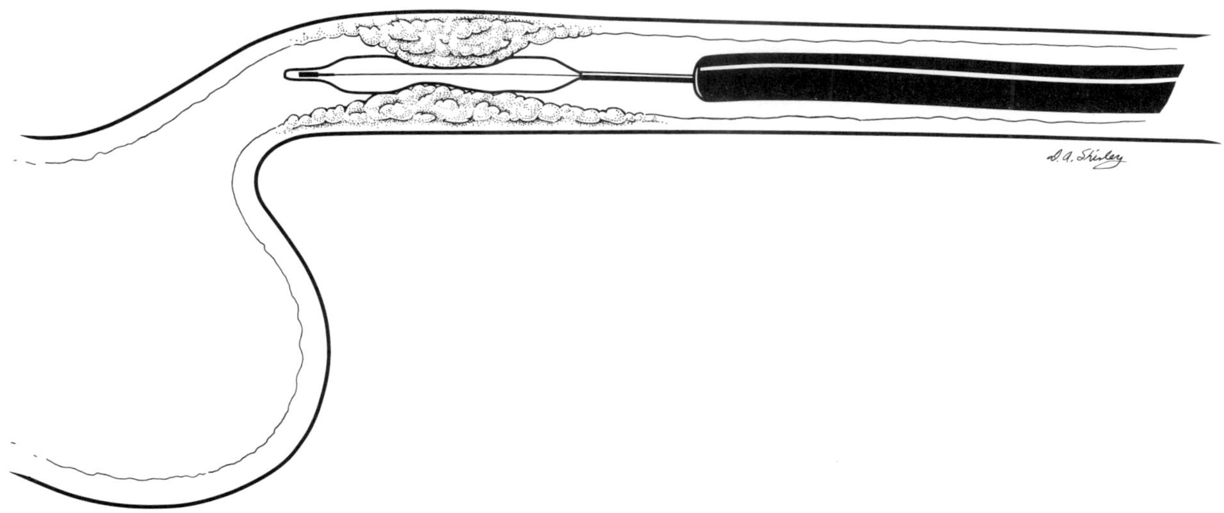

PLATE 5–2

After determining the length of the lesion, a stent of appropriate size is chosen and passed over the endoscope. A pusher tube is passed over the scope behind the prosthesis and a mark is made on the pusher tube at a distance from its tip equal to the distance of the top of the tumor to the patient's incisors. The distal end of the pusher tube is seated in the proximal end of the prosthesis and the entire complex is passed into the patient's esophagus **(A).**

The gastroscope is passed through the tumor and into the gastric lumen **(B).** The pusher tube is then advanced, pushing the prosthesis into the tumor channel, until the previously made mark on the pusher tube comes to rest at the patient's teeth. The top of the stent should now be positioned at the top of the tumor. This may be confirmed using fluoroscopy. The bottom flange of the prosthesis, which prevents it from riding up into the esophagus, should lie below the lesion.

A

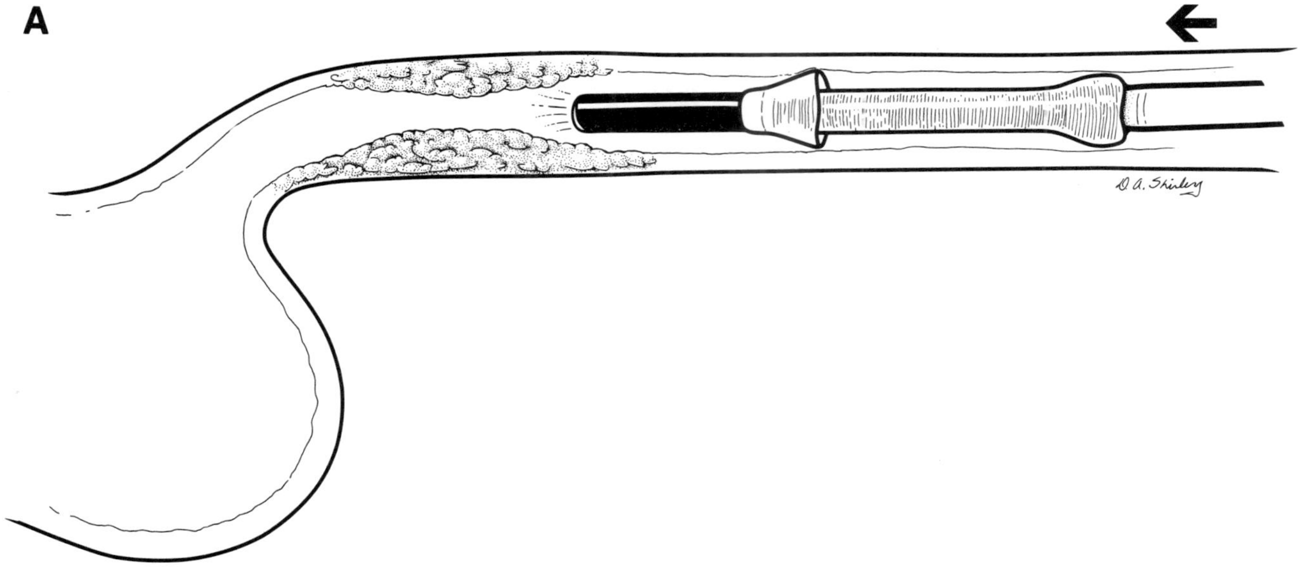

B

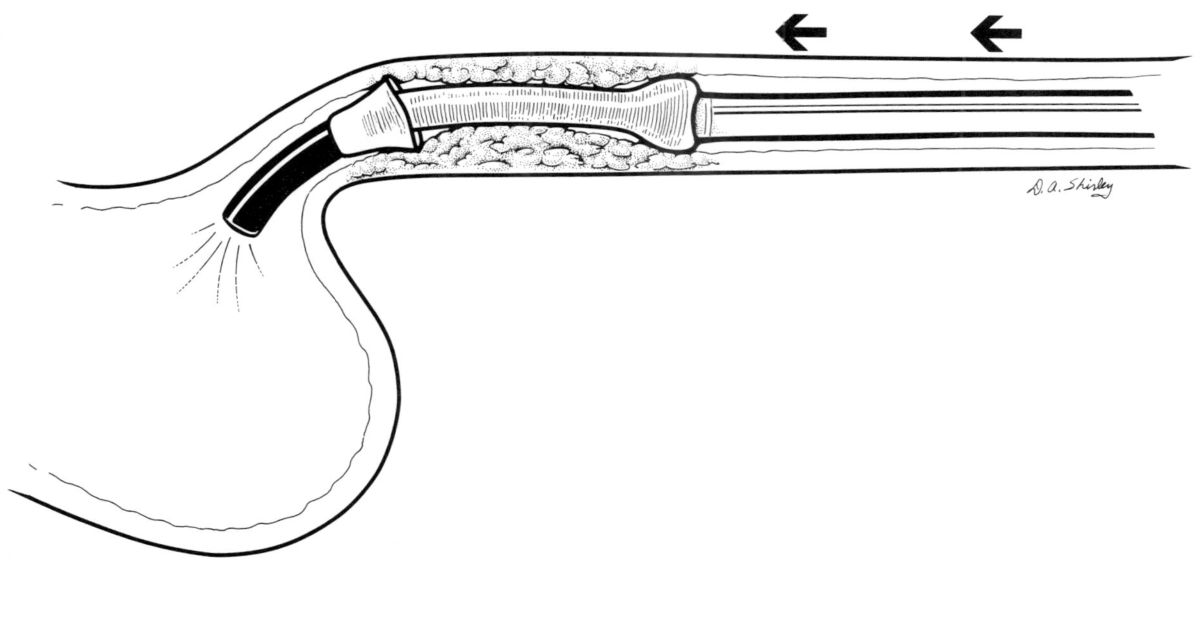

PLATE 5–3

After correct placement of the prosthesis is assured, the gastroscope and pusher tube may be withdrawn. A rim of the prosthesis should be visible above the tumor. Should the prosthesis be malpositioned, it may be adjusted or removed by use of a rat-toothed forceps or by inflation of the balloon at the distal end of the pusher tube.

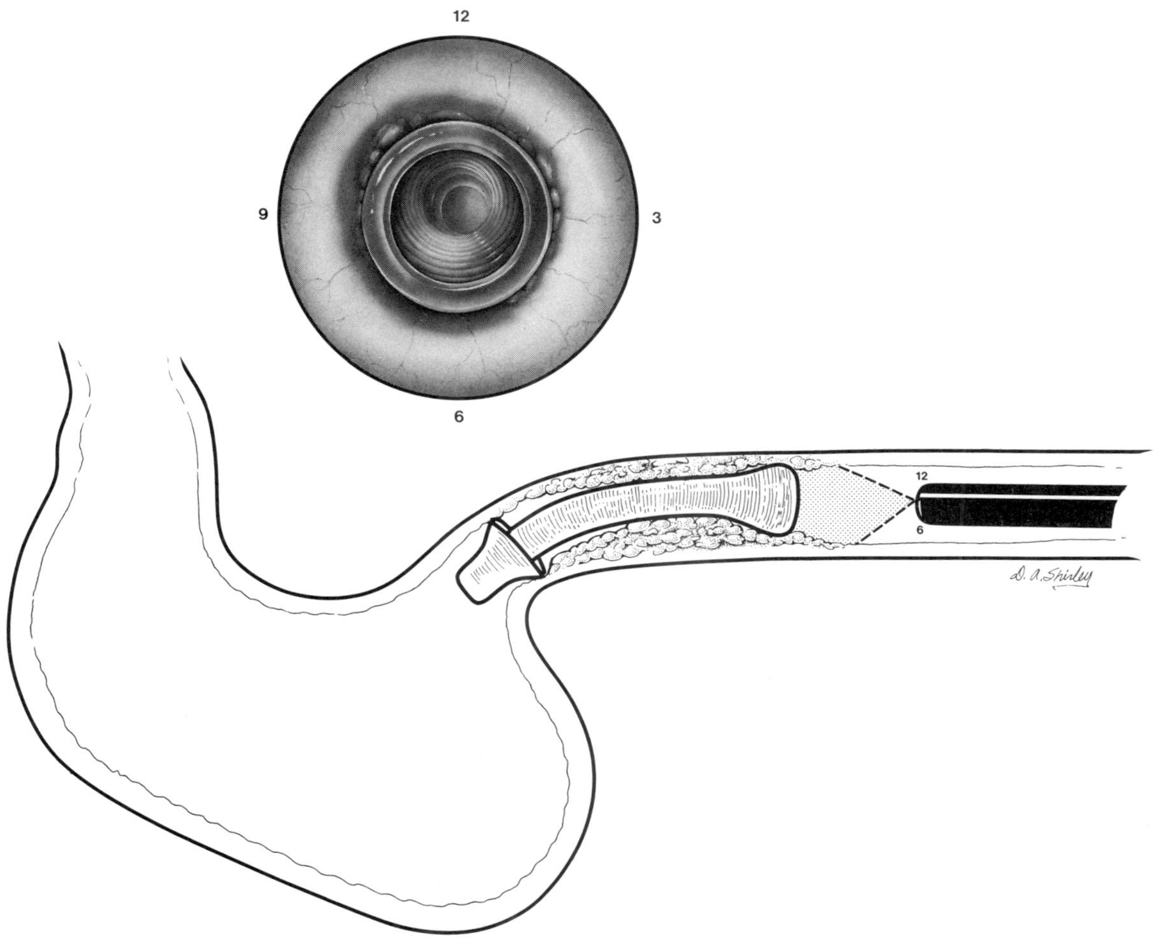
12
9
3
6
12
6

6

Retrieval of Foreign Bodies

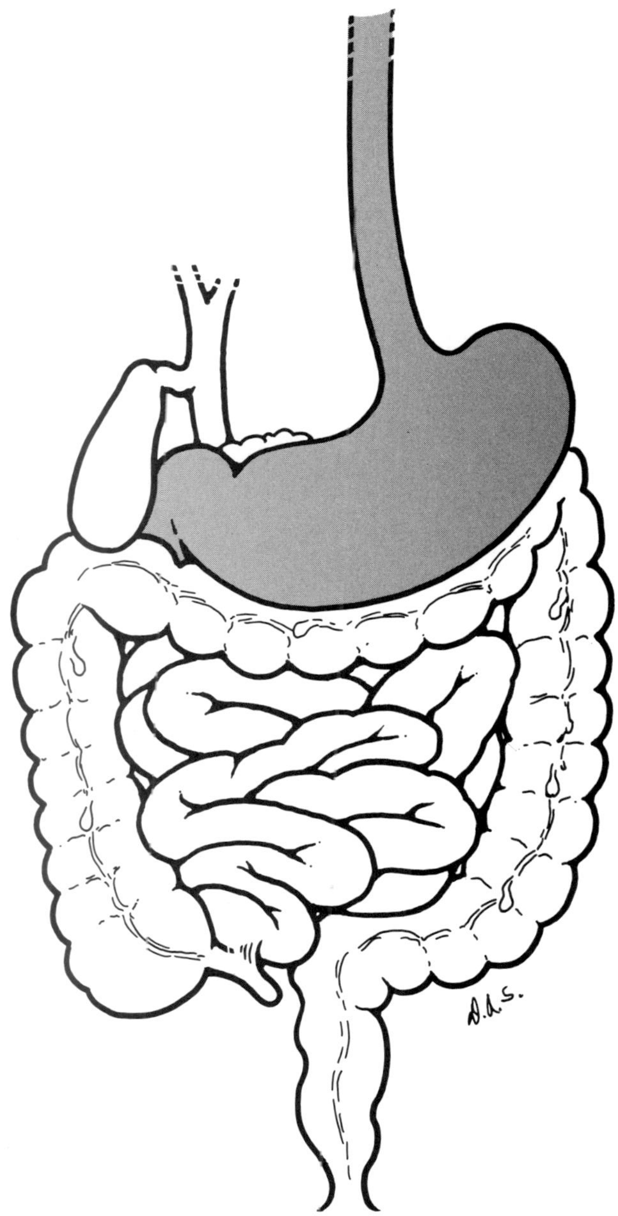

PLATE 6–1

Until two decades ago, foreign bodies of the gastrointestinal tract were best extracted with open-lumen rigid endoscopes or with surgery. Flexible endoscopic instrumentation and technique have progressed dramatically however, and currently, using long-established principles developed for rigid scopes and much ingenuity, almost all gastrointestinal foreign bodies within the reach of the flexible endoscope can be safely extracted.

Coins are frequently encountered foreign bodies in both children and adults. A lateral radiographic view may be helpful in distinguishing foreign bodies of the trachea from those in the esophagus. Small coins in the gastrointestinal tract may pass spontaneously, but those in the esophagus should be removed. Larger coins or other blunt objects may require extraction from the stomach. A variety of tools may be employed to grasp and remove foreign objects. A foreign body forceps with rubber jaws is often effective in grasping the edge of a coin. An alternate approach can be the use of a polypectomy snare applied around the waist of the coin.

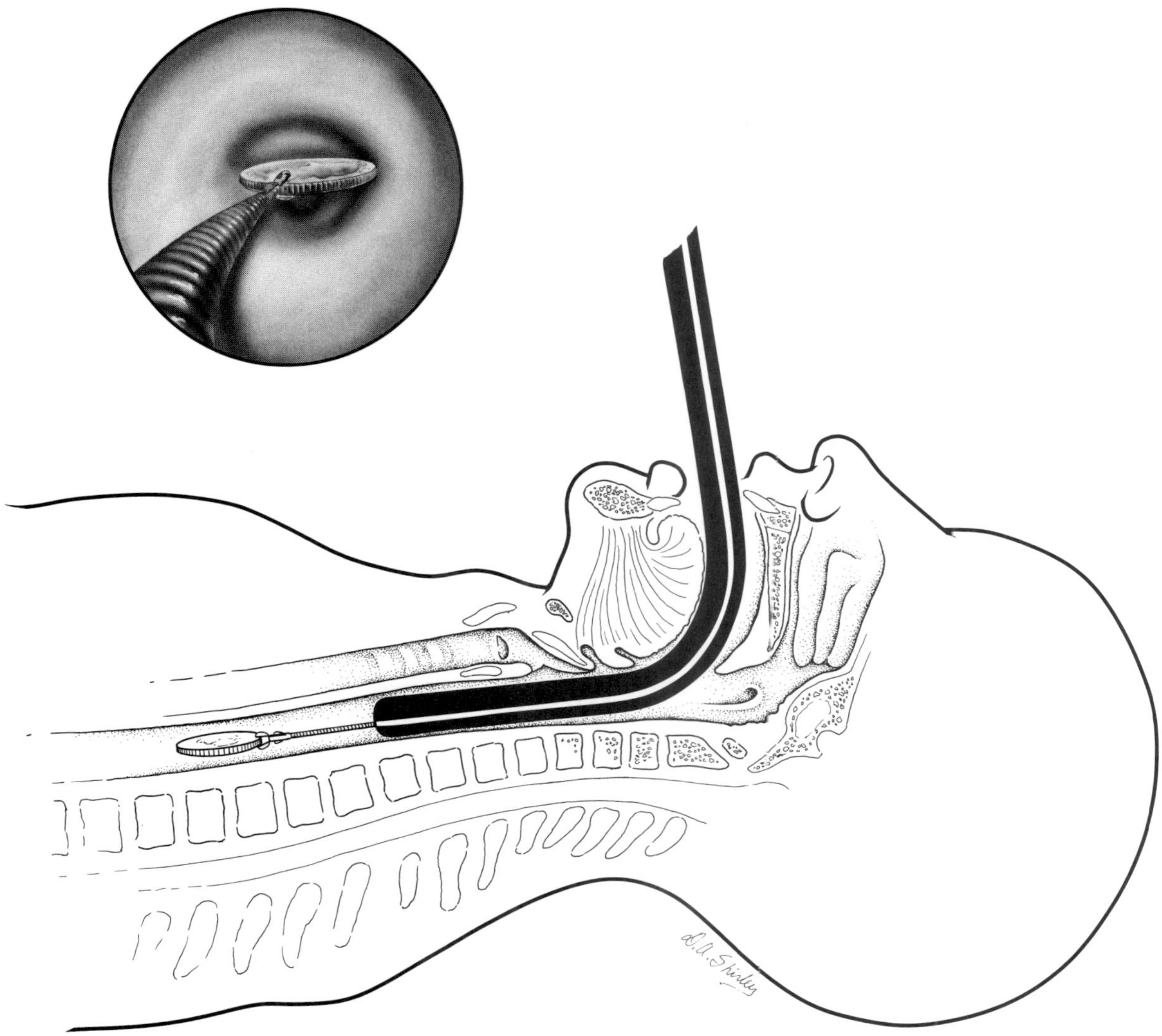

PLATE 6–2

Sharp foreign bodies such as pins or bones may come to lie in the esophagus with their tips pointing upward. Attempts to merely extract them may force the sharp points into the wall of the esophagus, creating a perforation.

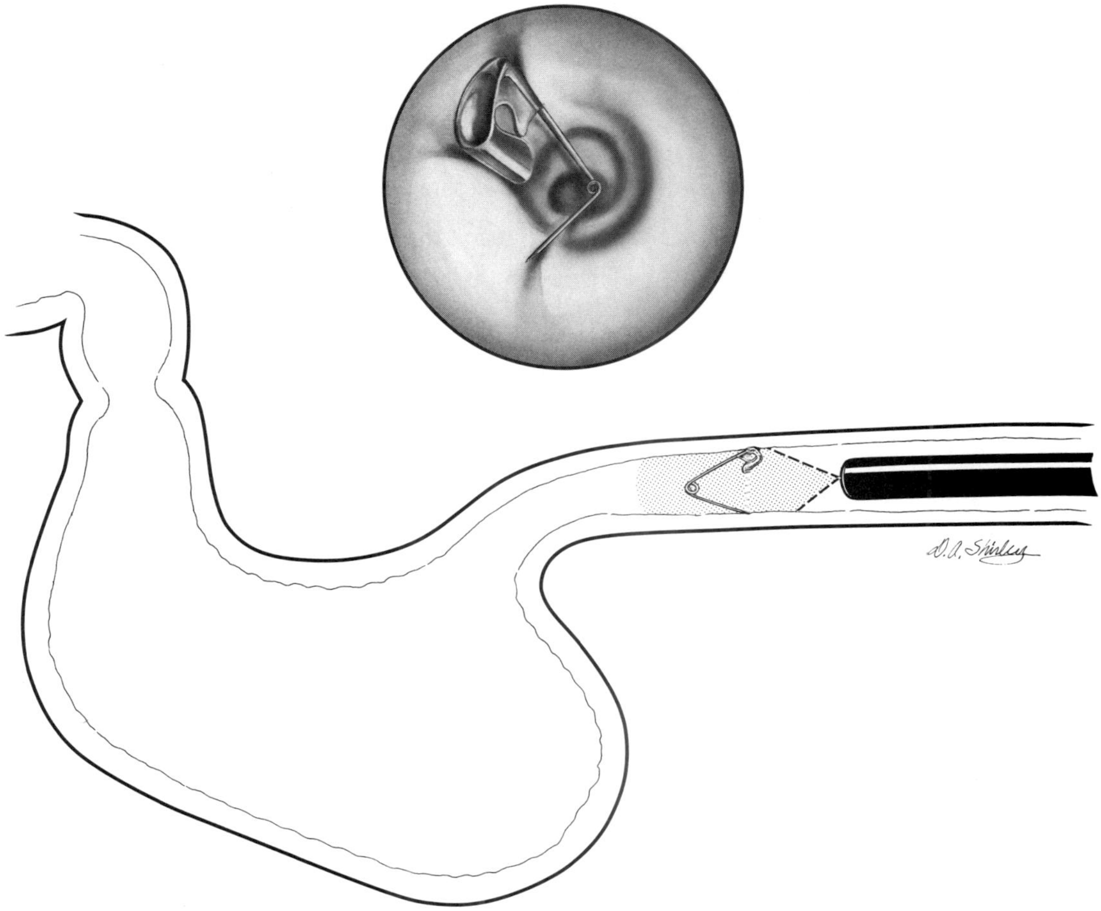

PLATE 6–3

The optimal approach for removing these articles is to grasp them with a forceps and advance them into the stomach for adjustment of their position **(A).** Once in the stomach, the article may be dropped and regrasped. A safety pin, as shown here, is grasped with a polypectomy snare opposite its points **(B).** Some manipulation of the article may be necessary to achieve this, but the gastric lumen is large and affords an adequate expanse for these maneuvers.

Once the snare has surrounded the foreign body, it is tightened around it at a position opposite the pointed end. The scope and foreign body are withdrawn together with the pointed end trailing **(C).** A trailing point is unlikely to cause perforation. Attempts to close the pin are usually unnecessary. When concern exists about injury to the esophageal wall, an overtube may be employed.

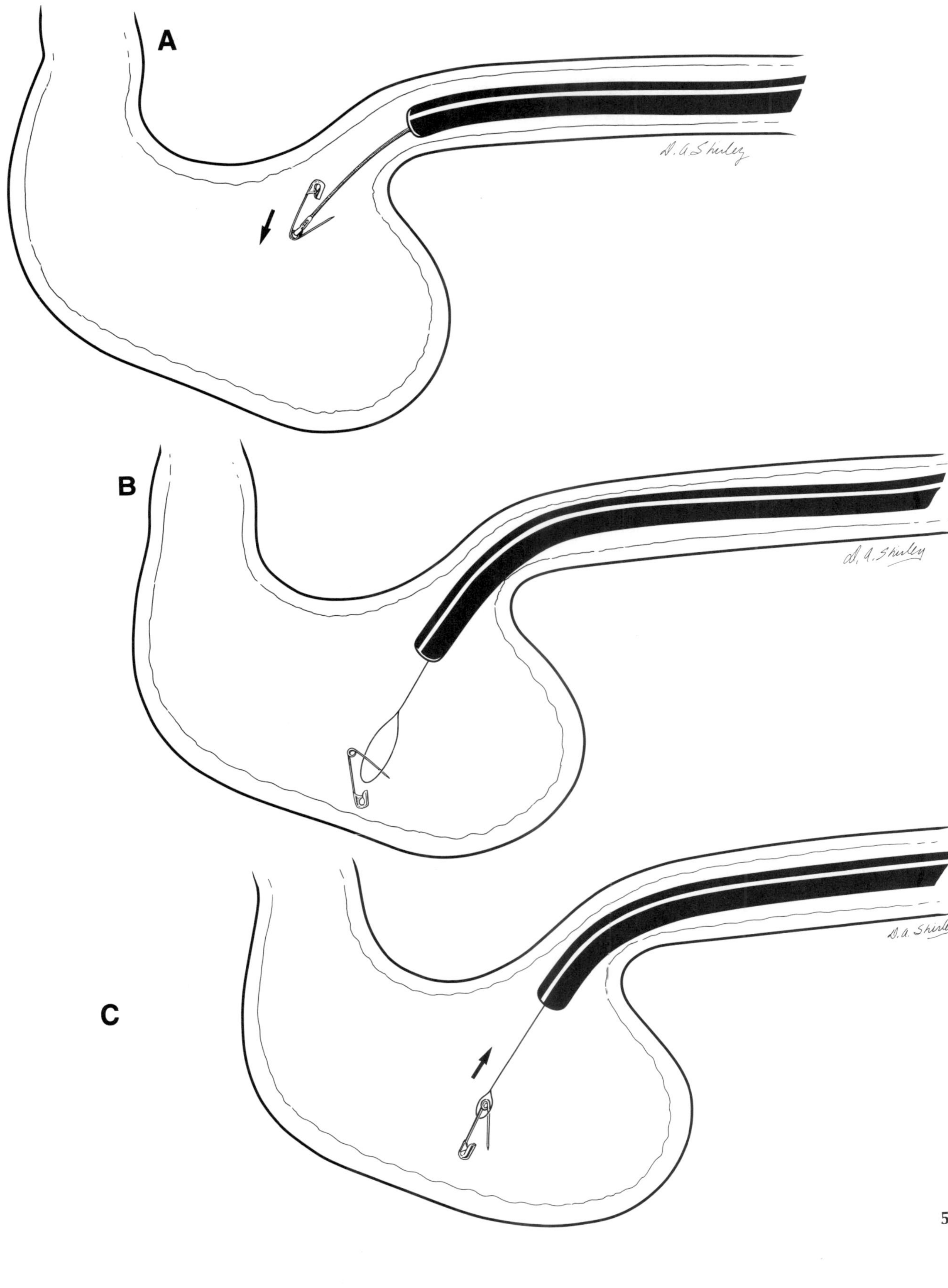
A
B
C

PLATE 6–4

Some foreign bodies, such as razor blades or glass, may have several sharp surfaces. These may be particularly likely to injure the esophagus if pulled through it. In such cases, the use of an overtube may prove the solution. Overtubes are constructed of flexible tubing and are loaded over the scope prior to its passage. The foreign body is grasped with a forceps and pulled up to the tip of the endoscope **(A).**

When the article has been firmly grasped, it is withdrawn into the overtube. If it is small, it may be extracted through the overtube. If larger, once it is well within the overtube, the entire scope-overtube complex may be removed **(B).**

Overtubes are particularly useful in removing multiple foreign bodies with a single passage of the scope. The overtube serves as a conduit for easy reinsertion of the instrument into the stomach without discomfort to the patient. It also protects the airway and prevents aspiration should the foreign body be dropped at the level of the vocal cords. (This method is also of value in retrieving gastric polyps following polypectomy.)

A

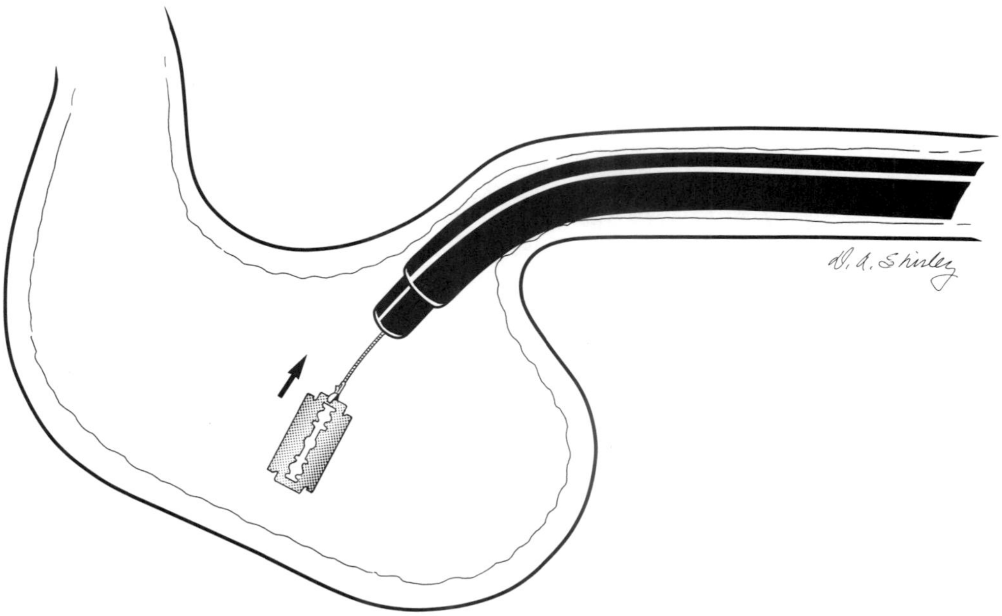

B

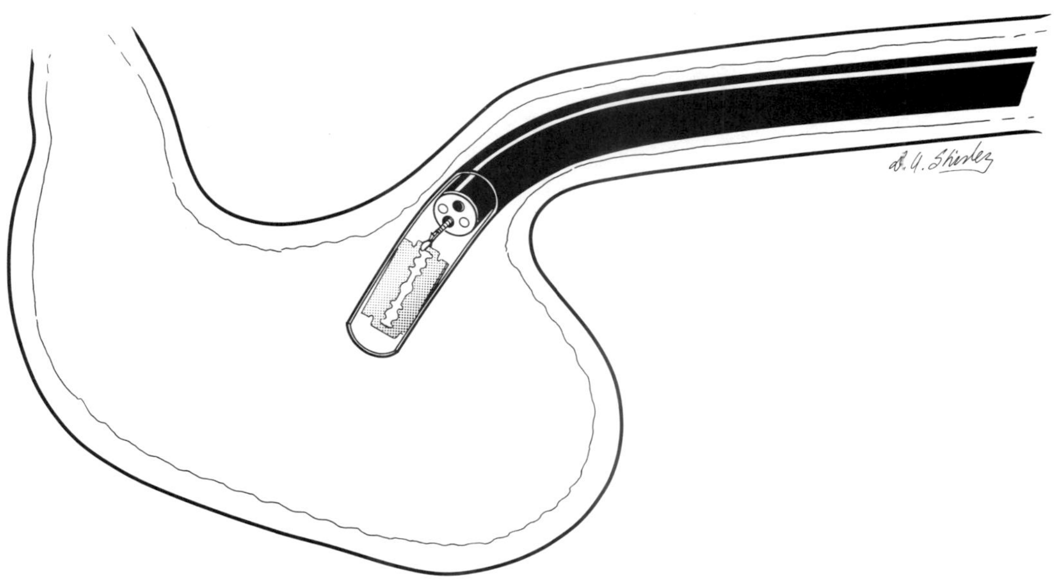

7

Percutaneous Endoscopic Gastrostomy

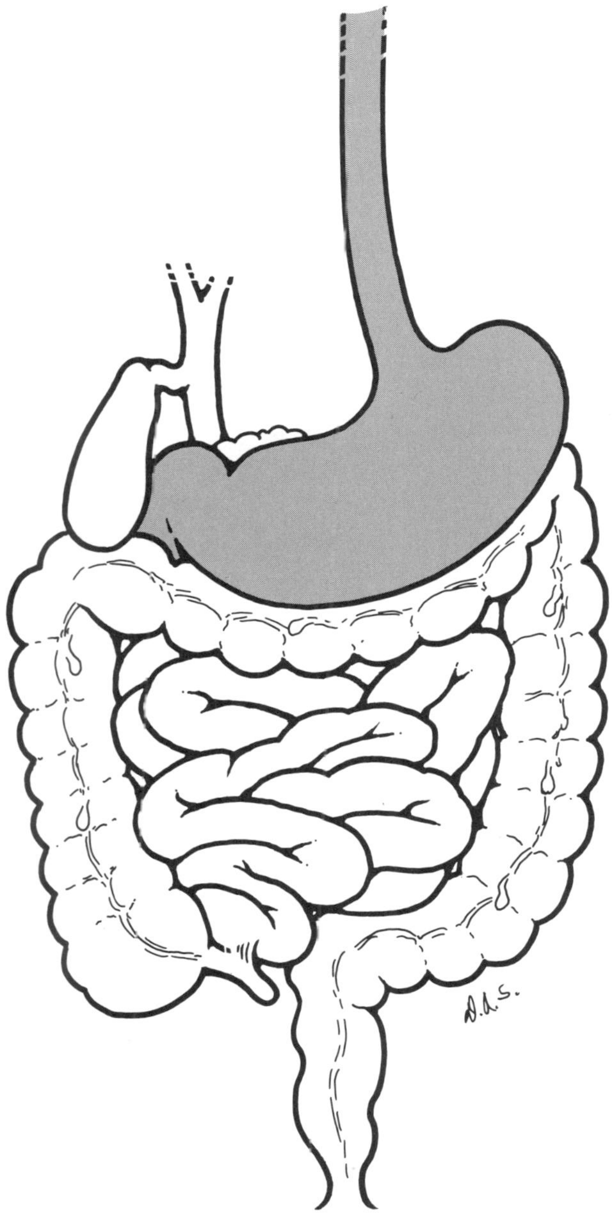

PLATE 7–1

Percutaneous endoscopic gastrostomy was introduced in 1980 as an alternative to traditional surgical gastrostomy. This technique permits the placement of a gastrostomy tube for feeding or decompression under endoscopic guidance, without the need for laparotomy or general anesthesia. Candidates for this procedure include adults and children with severe neurological impairment, patients with oropharyngeal neoplasms that impair swallowing or significant facial trauma, and those who need prolonged gastric decompression. Although a number of modifications of the technique have been described, the pull method (shown here) is the most widely used.

With the patient in the supine position, the endoscope is passed into the stomach. The stomach is inflated and the room lights dimmed so that the light of the gastroscope transilluminates the abdominal wall. An assistant prepares the abdominal wall using an antiseptic solution and applies finger pressure at the point at which he notes transillumination is best. This indicates contact of the gastric and abdominal walls without intervening tissue. Finger pressure applied to the abdominal wall at this site should produce a distinctive bulge within the gastric lumen as observed by the endoscopist.

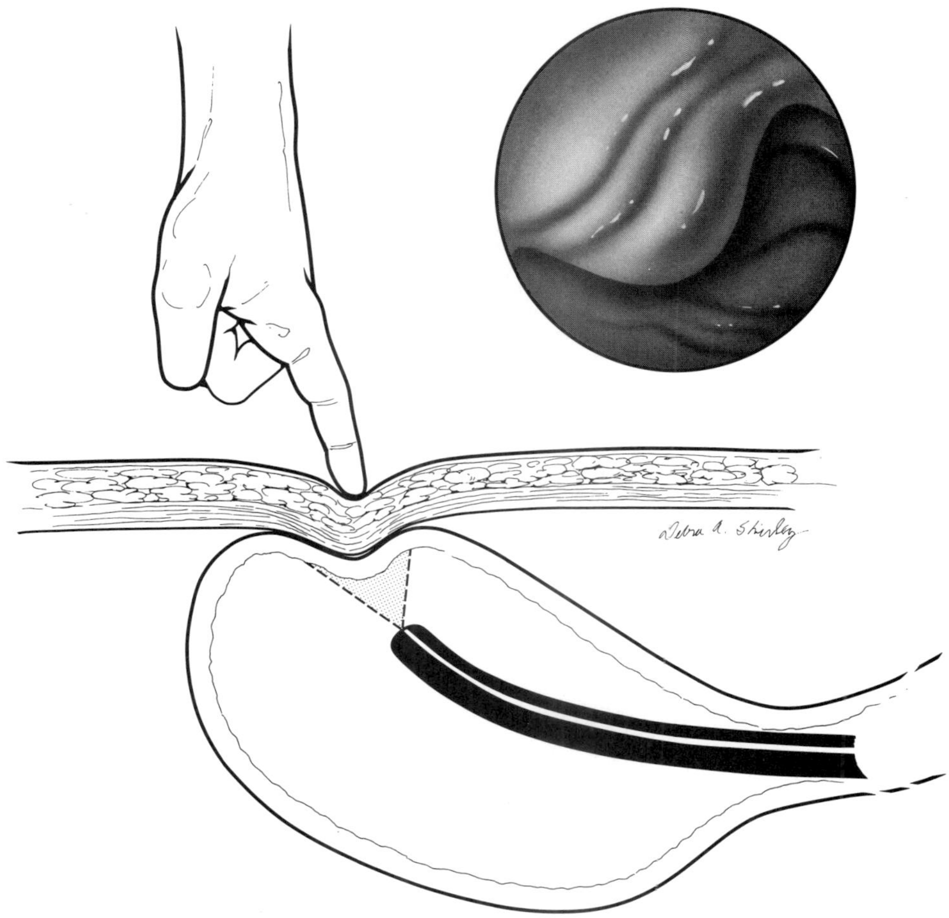

PLATE 7–2

The endoscopist passes a polypectomy snare through the biopsy channel of the endoscope and opens it over the indentation of the gastric wall produced by the assistant's finger pressure.

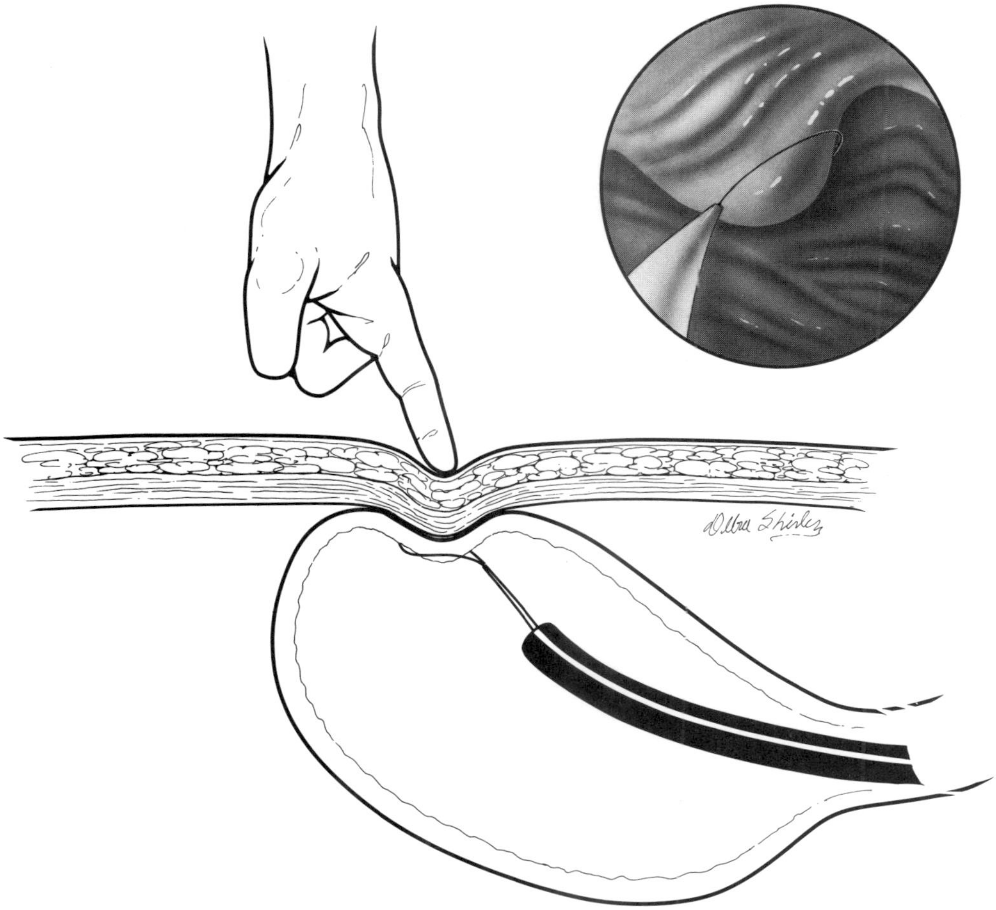

PLATE 7–3

A 1-cm skin incision is made at the selected point and an intravenous cannula is thrust across the opposed gastric and abdominal walls into the gastric lumen. The snare is tightened down around the cannula and the inner stylet of the cannula is then removed. A loop of coated wire suture is then passed through the cannula until the endoscopist sees it appear inside the stomach.

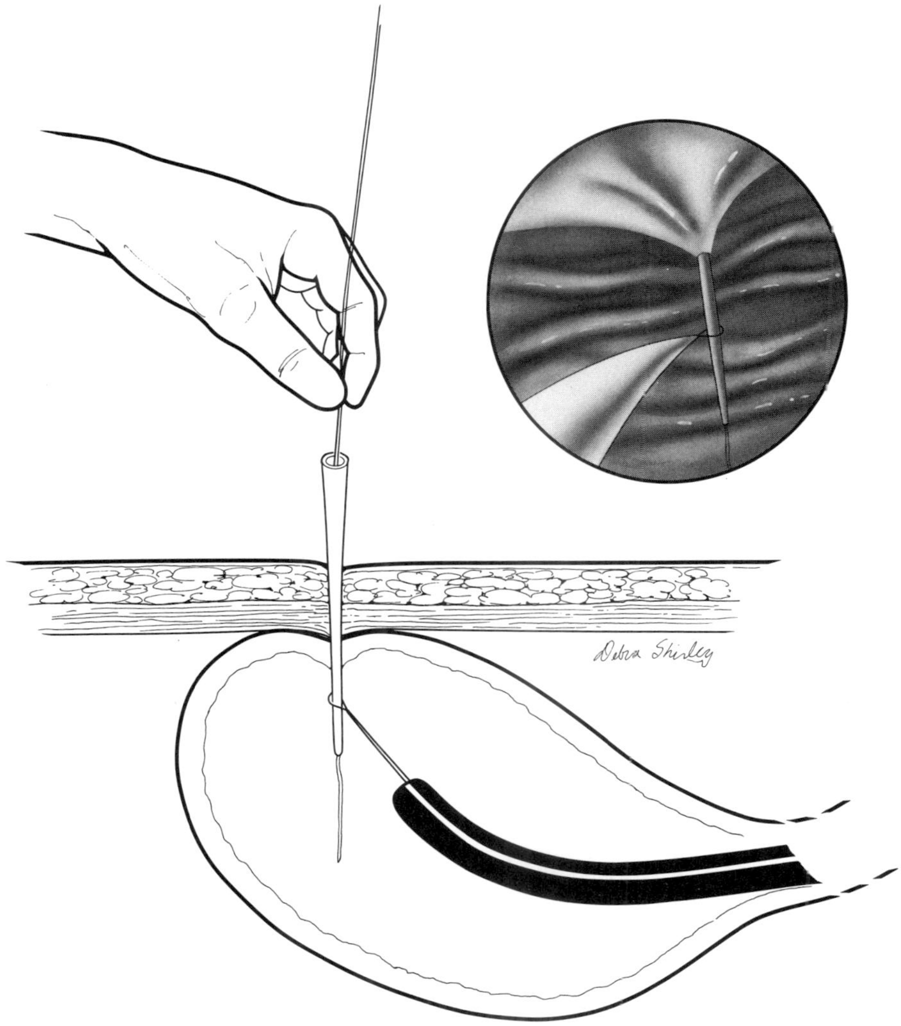
Debra Shirley

PLATE 7–4

After several inches of suture have emerged from the cannula and appeared in the gastric lumen, the snare is loosened, the cannula pulled slightly back, and the snare retightened around the suture itself. The scope and suture are then pulled up the esophagus and out of the patient's mouth.

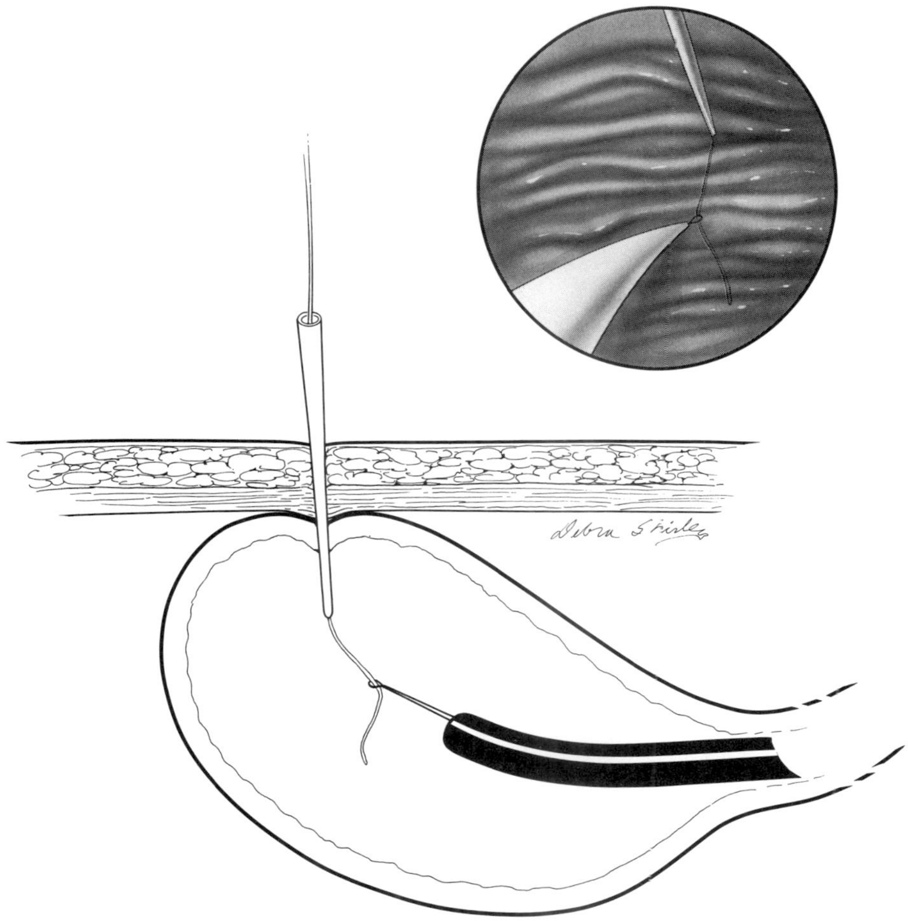

PLATE 7–5

The suture emerging from the patient's mouth is tied to the tapered end of the gastrostomy tube. The assistant begins pulling on the abdominal end of the suture and the tube is pulled into the patient's esophagus. The gastroscope is again inserted to follow the gastrostomy tube into the stomach and assure its correct positioning.

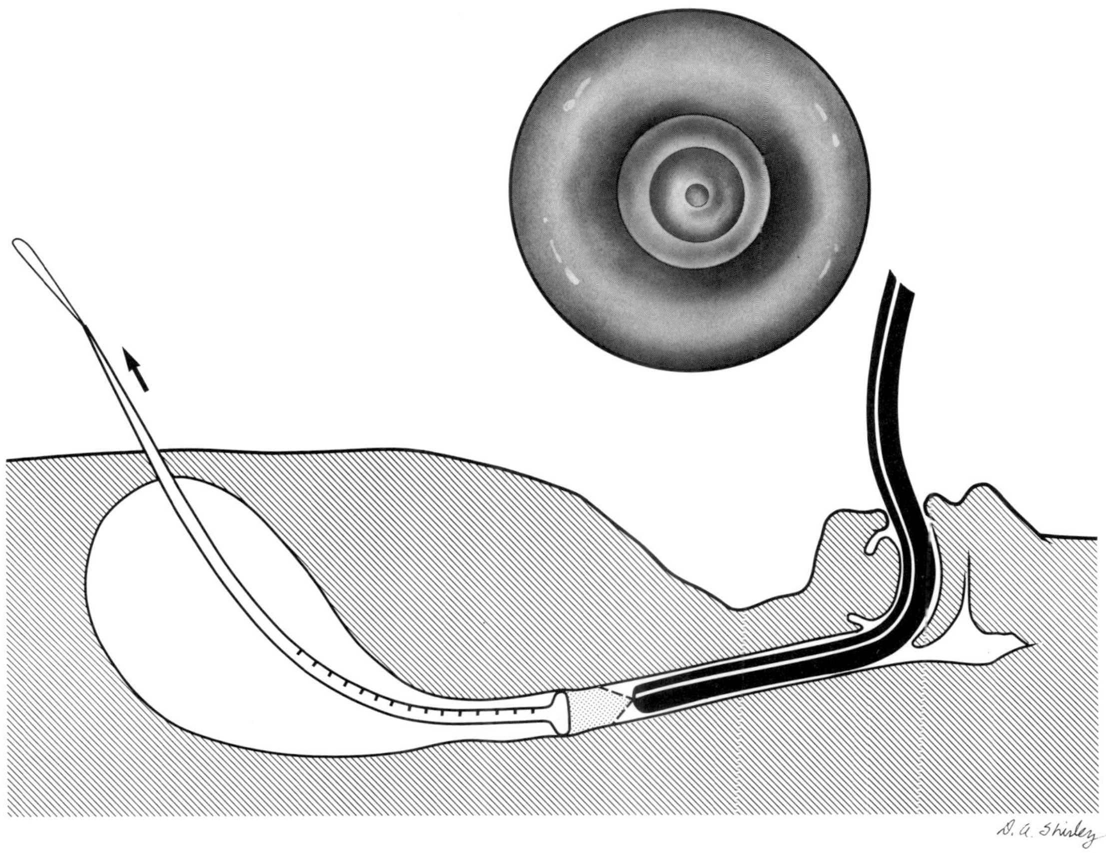

PLATE 7–6

The tube is pulled into the stomach until its mushroom-shaped head lightly touches the gastric mucosa. Tension on the tube should be avoided as it produces ischemia of the underlying tissue with risk of subsequent necrosis, infection, or extrusion of the tube. Only slight tissue contact between the stomach serosa and the peritoneal surface is desirable and sufficient for adhesion.

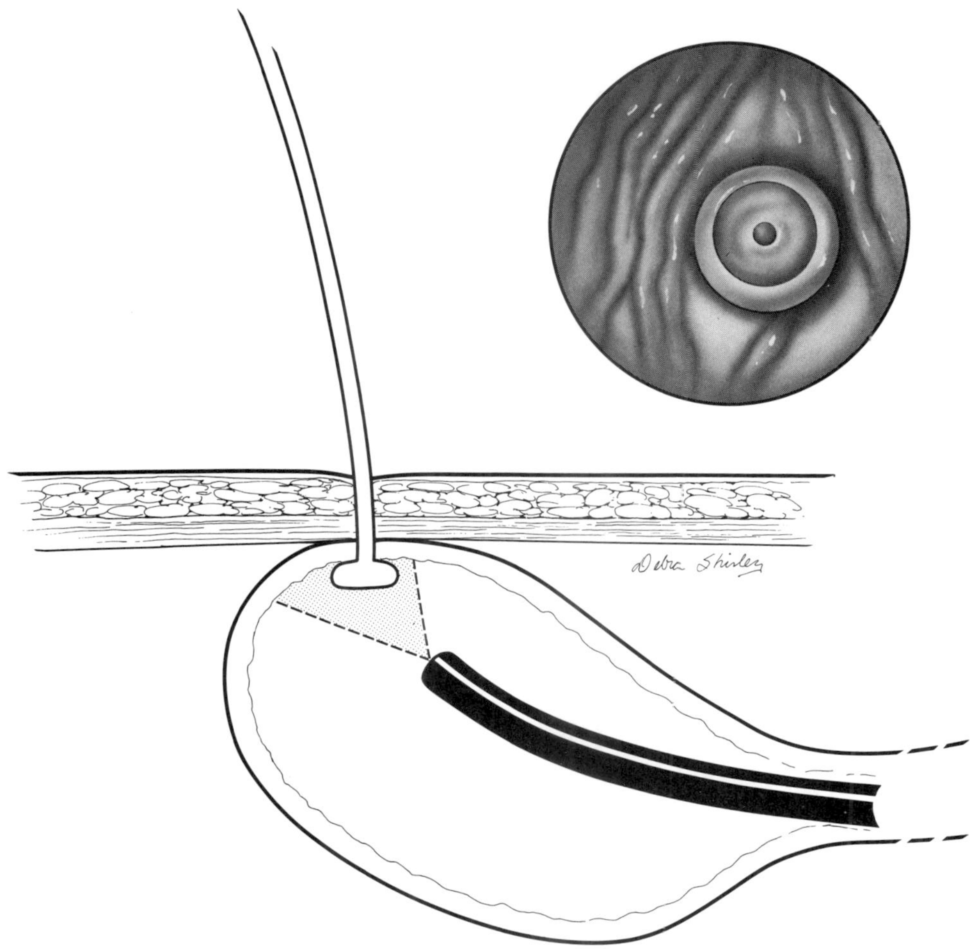

PLATE 7–7

An outer crossbar is applied loosely on the external portion of the tube in order to prevent migration inward. Sutures or an O-ring may be affixed to the tube to prevent dislodgement.

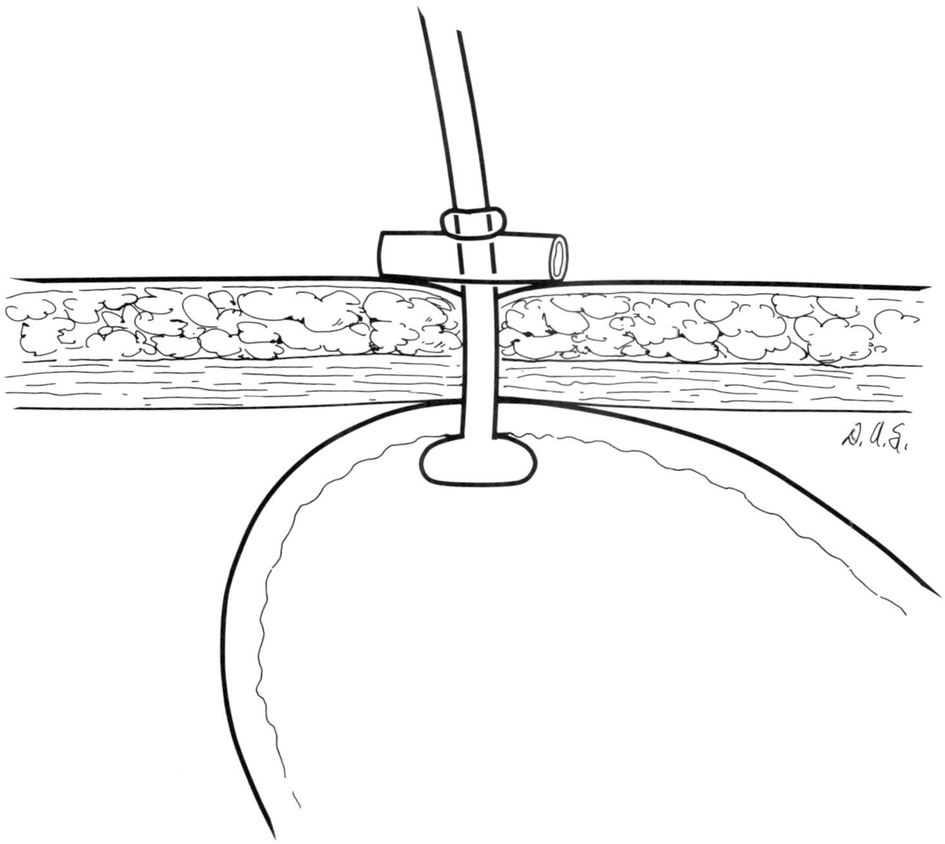
D.A.G.

8

Control of Upper Gastrointestinal Tract Bleeding

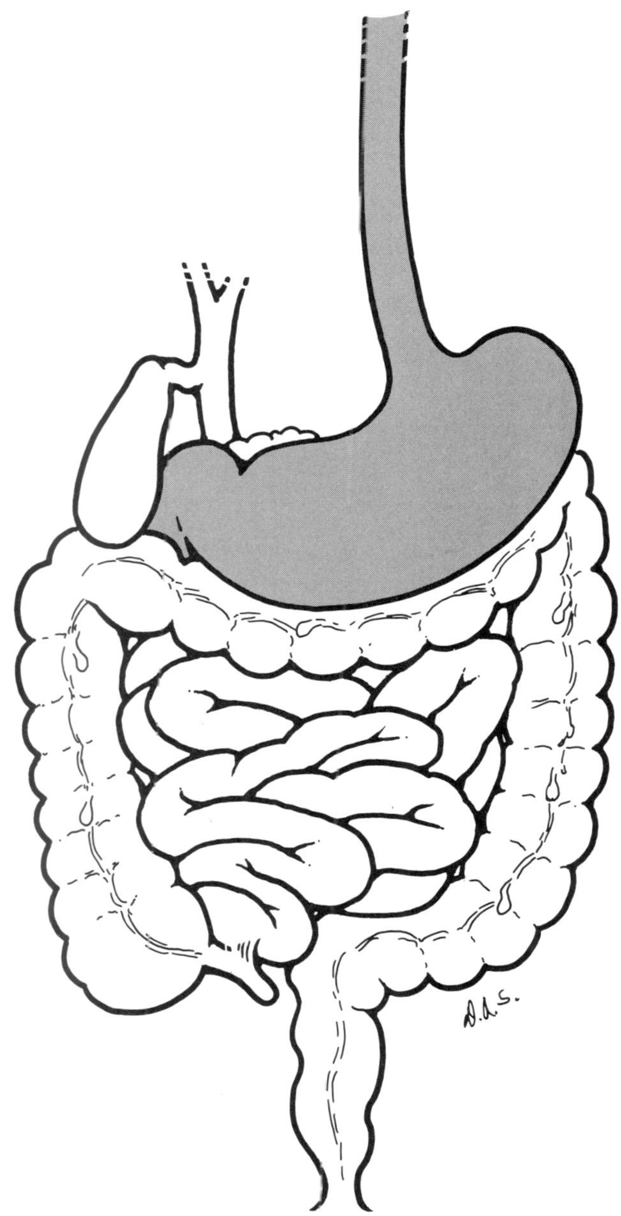

PLATE 8–1

Bleeding from the upper gastrointestinal tract is a common indication for endoscopic examination. The patient must be resuscitated and his condition stabilized prior to any attempts at endoscopic diagnosis or therapy. When acute hemorrhage is present, the stomach fills with clotted blood, which obscures vision and precludes an adequate endoscopic examination. Prior to endoscopic examination of the patient with acute bleeding, therefore, it is necessary to pass a large-bore tube, such as an Ewald tube, into which extra holes have been cut. Irrigation is then vigorously carried out with room-temperature tap water in order to disrupt and remove clotted blood **(A).** Use of a smaller-caliber tube is unlikely to cleanse the stomach adequately.

Removal of clot from the stomach by irrigation permits direct visualization of the bleeding lesion **(B)** and affords an opportunity for therapy. Frequently the bleeding has ceased by the time the examination is performed.

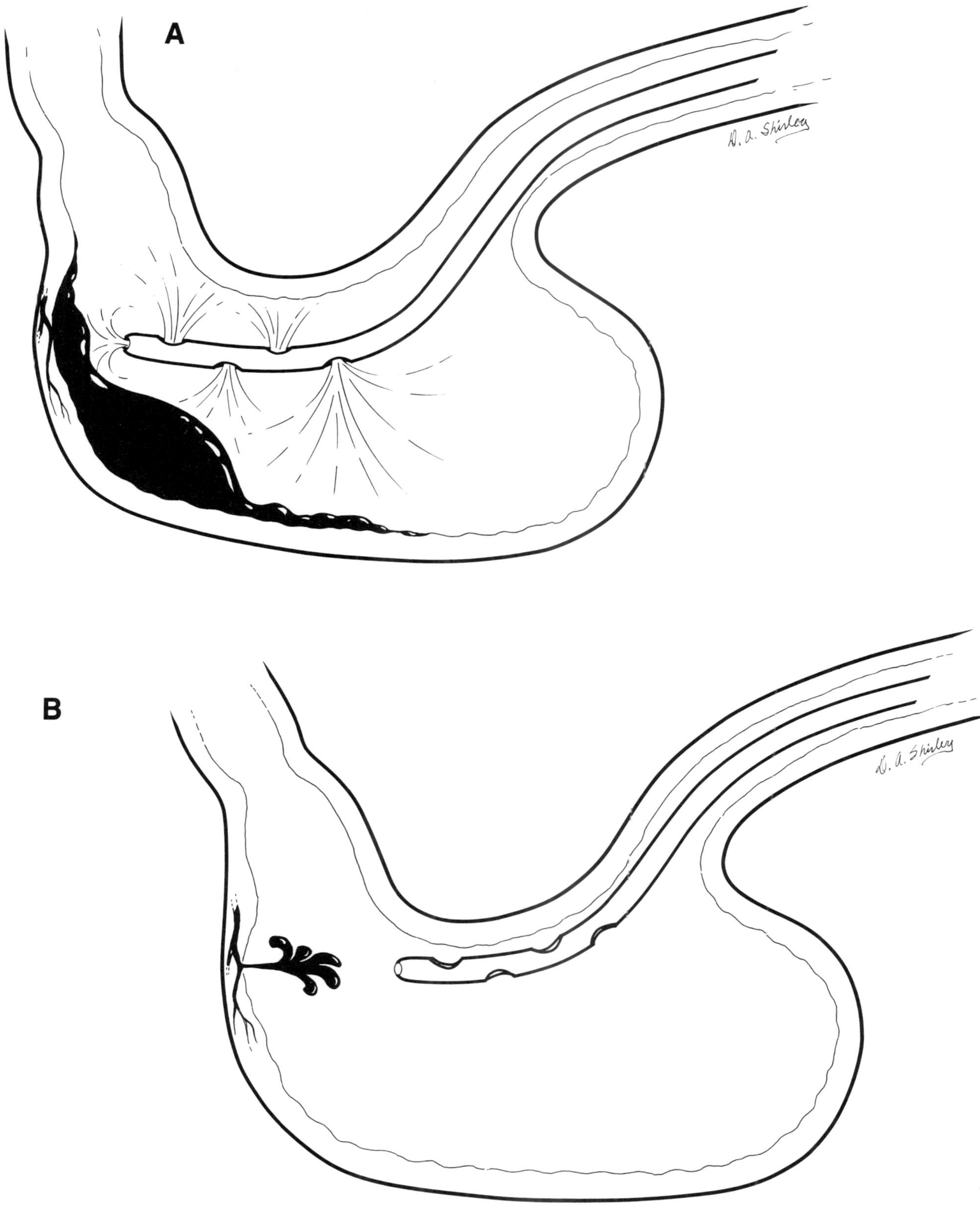
A
B

PLATE 8–2

After removal of clot from the stomach, the endoscope is introduced and the stomach systematically examined. An ulcer is often the source of the bleeding episode. Duodenal and prepyloric ulcers are most common. The ulcer appears as a crater with heaped-up mucosa at its edges. If a nonbleeding ulcer is identified and no vessel is obvious at its base, it is usually best left undisturbed; however, ulcers that demonstrate the appearance of a vessel at their base (a visible vessel or a pigmented protuberance) are very likely to bleed again. When such lesions are found, endoscopic therapy may be employed. The visible vessel may actually represent the eroded side of a blood vessel, rather than its end.

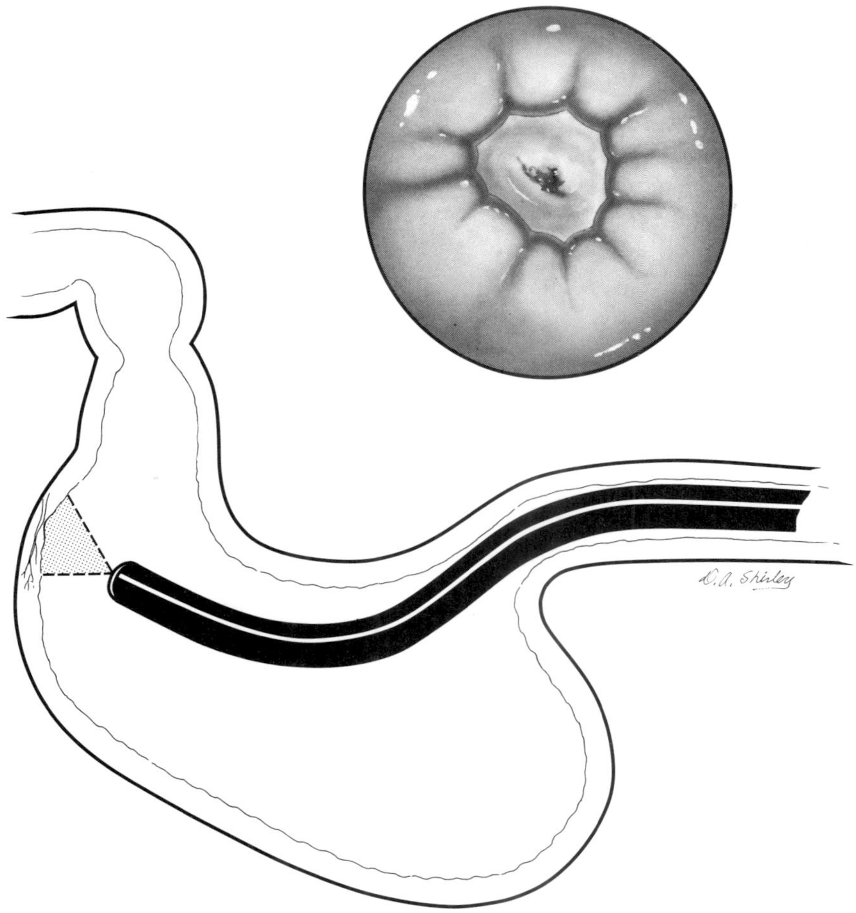

PLATE 8–3

Therapy may be delivered by means of a monopolar or bipolar electrocoagulation device, a heater probe, laser energy, or injection. This plate demonstrates the method in which a bipolar probe is used to coagulate an ulcer base. Current is applied in a circumferential pattern around the central vessel to obliterate vascular channels going into and out of the bleeding site. The central area may then be coagulated, if necessary. The method is similar for monopolar and bipolar coagulation, although monopolar current is less predictable. Laser energy is used in a similar fashion.

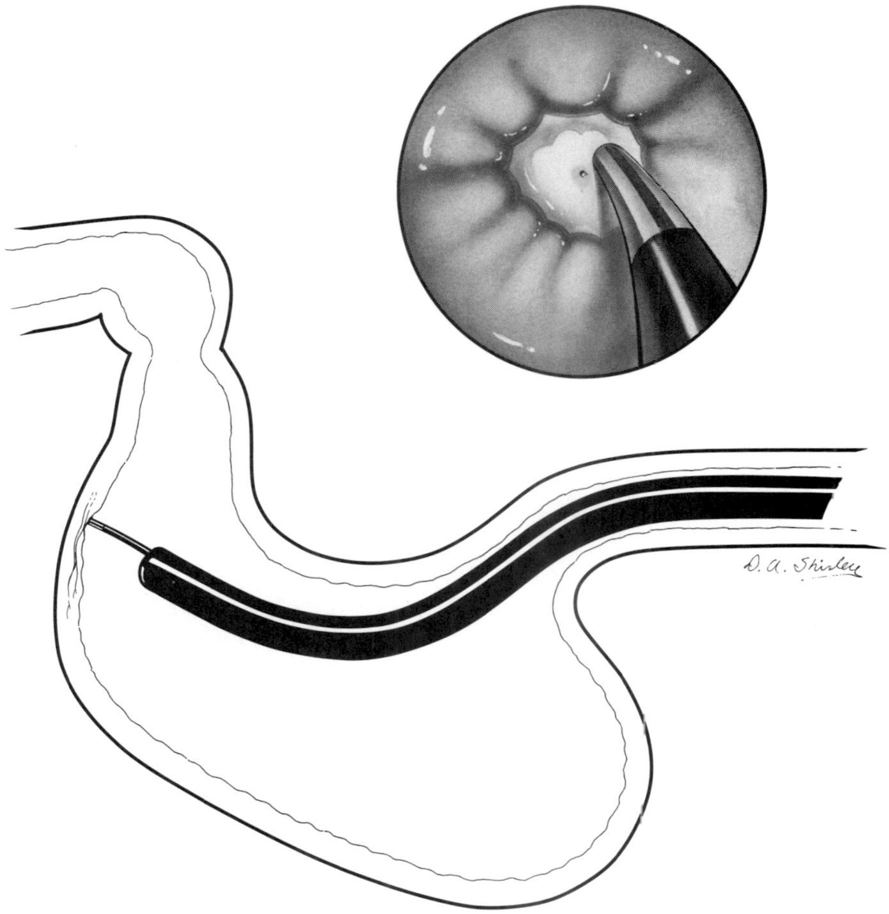

PLATE 8–4

The heater probe is applied, with pressure, directly to the center of the lesion in an attempt to coapt and seal the bleeding vessel.

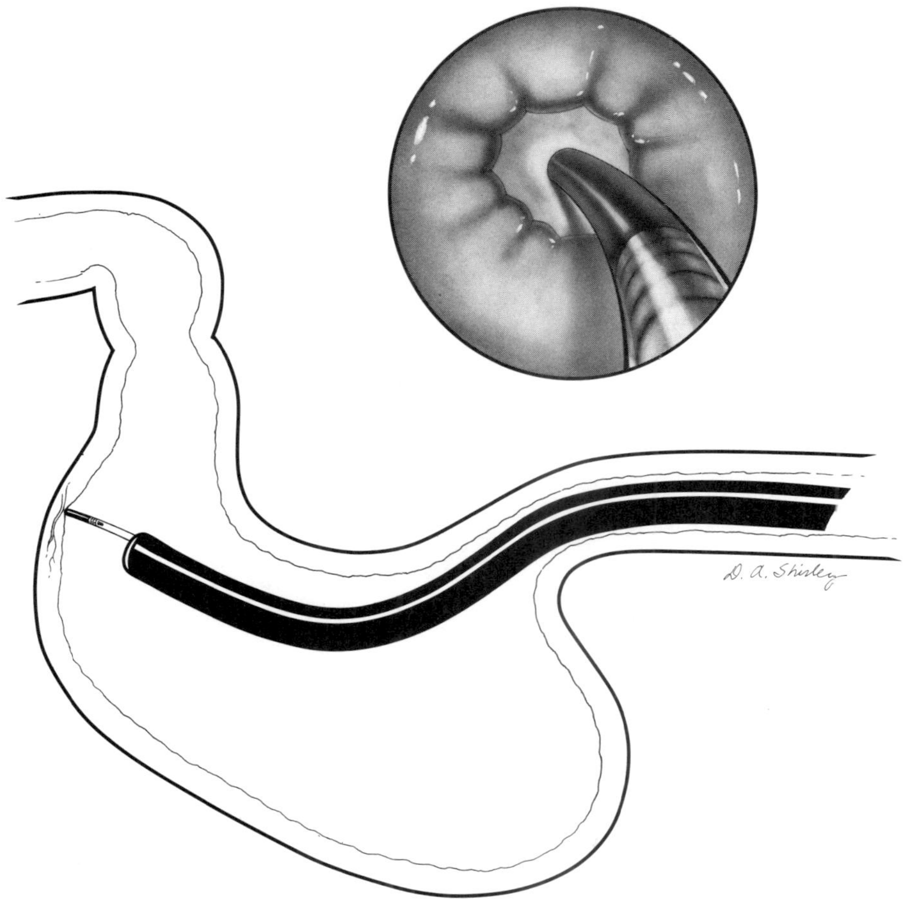
D. A. Shirley

PLATE 8–5

Injection of solutions of epinephrine (1:10,000) alone or in combination with sclerosants may be extremely effective in achieving control of gastrointestinal hemorrhage, particularly when a direct view of the bleeding site is difficult to obtain. Injection is performed circumferentially around the bleeding lesion to produce vasospasm and tissue edema.

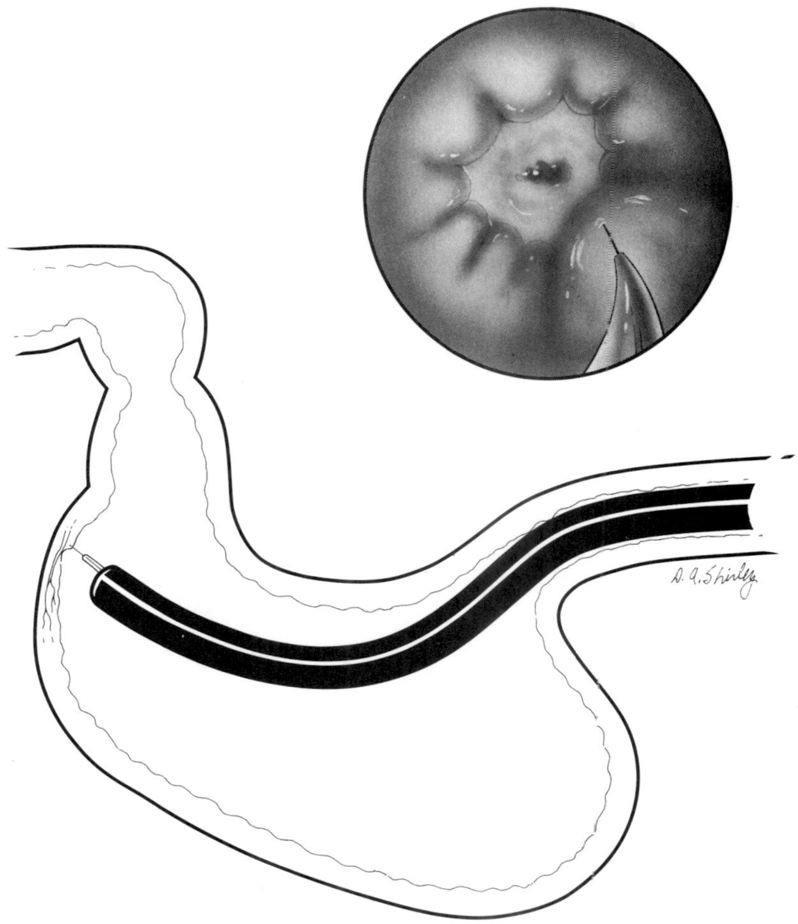

PLATE 8–6

Laser energy may be delivered through the endoscope to control hemorrhage. The Nd-YAG (neodymium: yttrium-aluminum-garnet) laser has been most effective. The laser energy is applied around the circumference of the lesion first, treating the central area last. High cost, lack of portability, and equally effective alternative methods have decreased the use of lasers in the treatment of upper gastrointestinal hemorrhage.

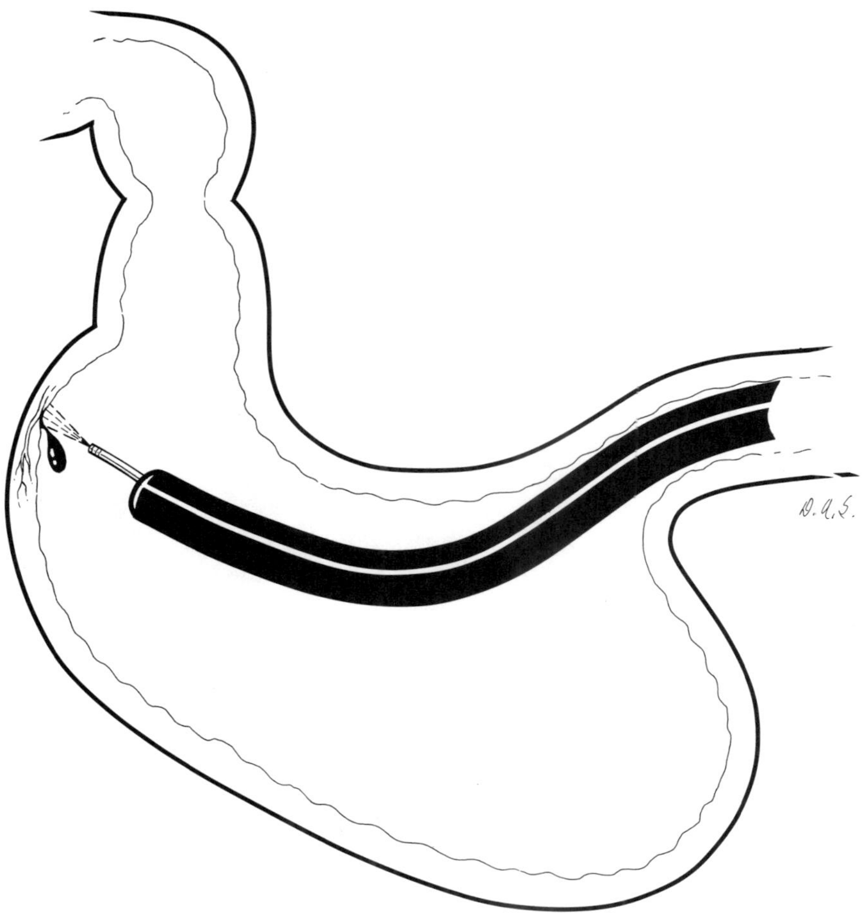

9

Endoscopic Retrograde Cholangiopancreatography (ERCP)

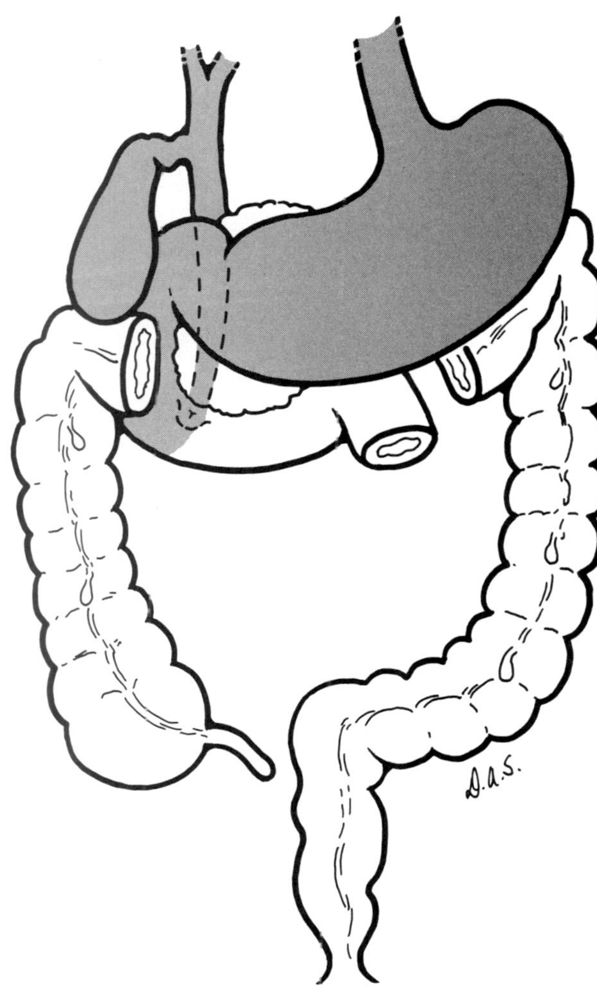

PLATE 9–1

ERCP is an endoscopic procedure designed to obtain an x-ray image of the anatomy of the biliary and pancreatic ductal systems. It must be performed in a suite with fluoroscopic capability. Indications for the procedure include suspected abnormalities of the biliary and pancreatic systems, benign and malignant. In many cases endoscopic therapy may follow confirmation of a diagnosis.

The instrument utilized for ERCP is a side-viewing duodenoscope, which is somewhat longer than the standard gastroduodenoscope. Its focal length is short, as it is designed to provide optimal visualization of the ampulla of Vater. The instrument is advanced into the stomach. The view demonstrated in this plate is that seen as the scope comes to rest in the gastric antrum. The endoscopist will see both the antrum and pylorus ahead, as well as the cardia above. This view is a useful landmark and indicates that the instrument's tip should now be directed downward and advanced toward the pylorus.

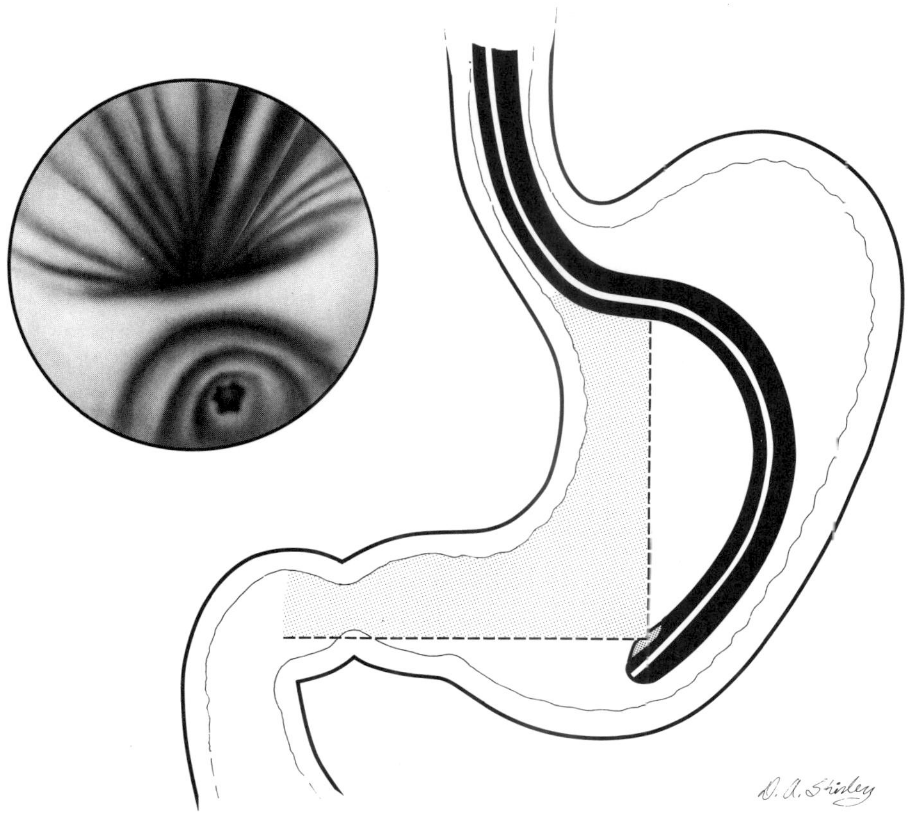

PLATE 9–2

As the pylorus is approached, it will be necessary for the operator to direct the instrument's tip downward in order to maintain the pylorus in the center of the visual field.

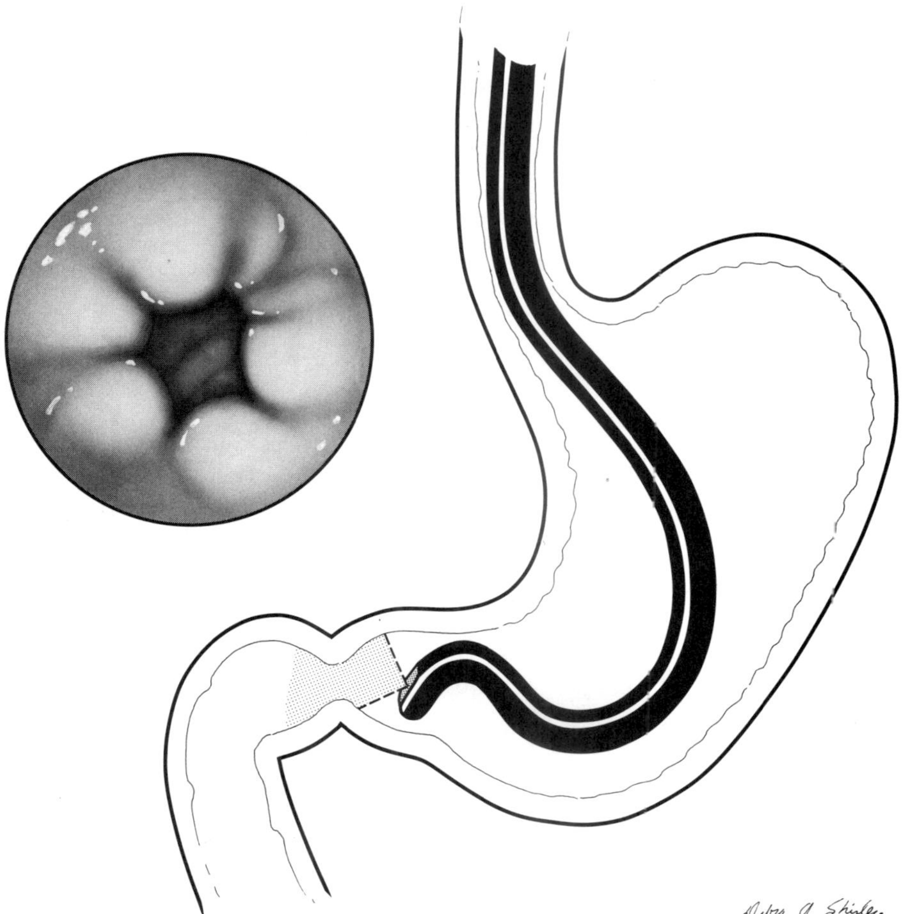

PLATE 9–3

In order to pass the duodenoscope through the pylorus, the endoscopist must raise the tip of the instrument. The pylorus will disappear from view at the 6 o'clock position. Pressure is applied as the tip is raised. The instrument's tip will be seen and felt to "pop" through the pylorus into the duodenal bulb.

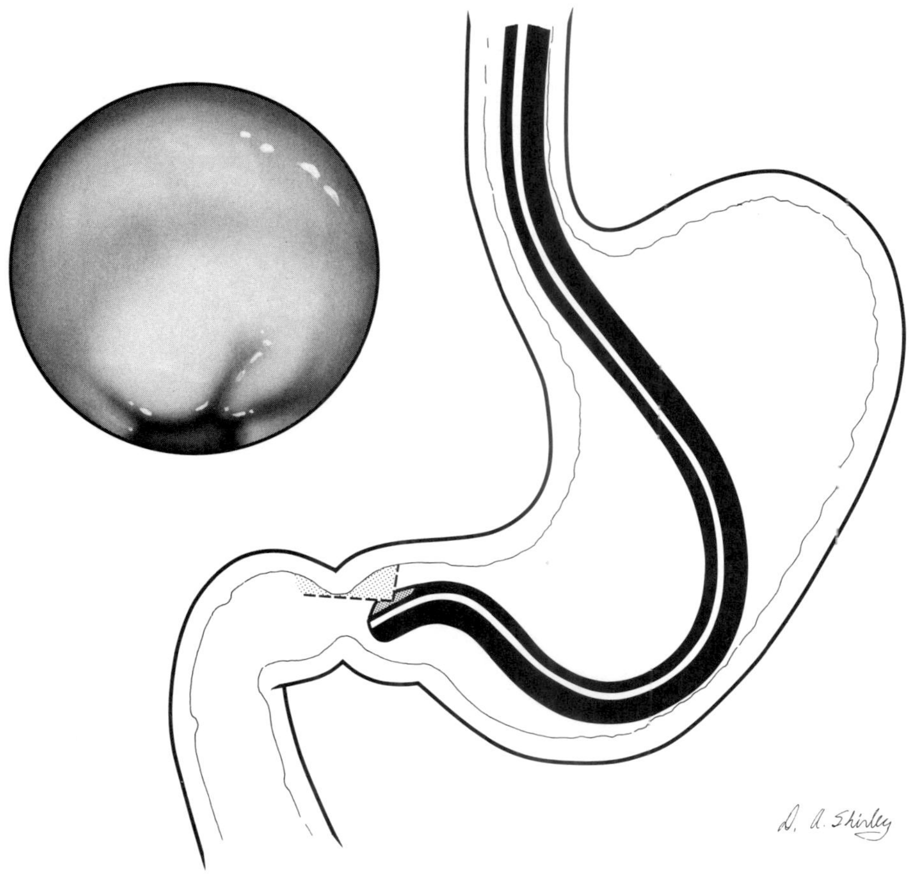

PLATE 9–4

Once in the duodenal bulb, the tip of the instrument is lowered slightly to observe the lumen. The scope is advanced slightly and its tip is then directed upward and posteriorly (to the right). This maneuver will direct the instrument into the descending portion of the duodenum.

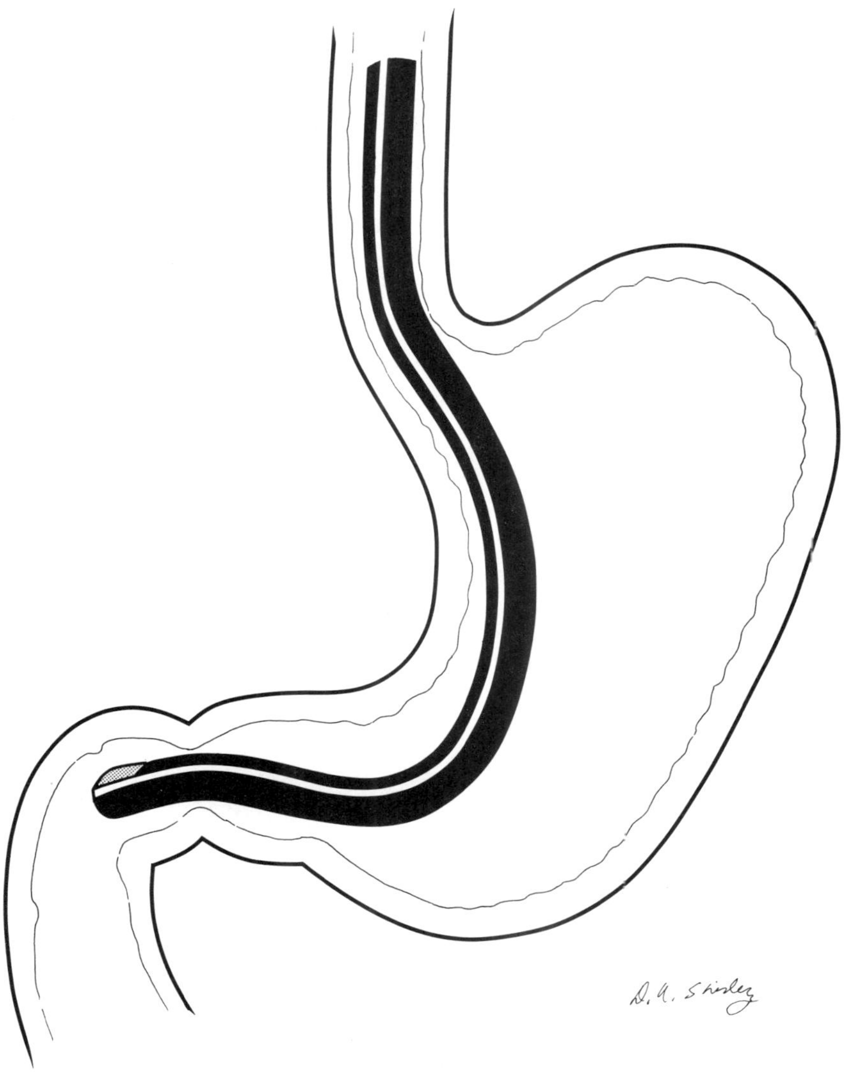
D. A. Shirley

PLATE 9–5

Once the duodenoscope is in the descending duodenum, the endoscopist should carefully search for the ampulla of Vater. At this point in the procedure the instrument is in its long position along the greater curvature of the stomach; this can be confirmed with fluoroscopy. The ampulla of Vater often appears in the 10 o'clock position. Frequently, a smaller, accessory papilla may be seen more proximal to and to the right of the ampulla of Vater. It is useful to turn the patient to the prone position at this point in the procedure; this will rotate the ampulla more toward the 12 o'clock position.

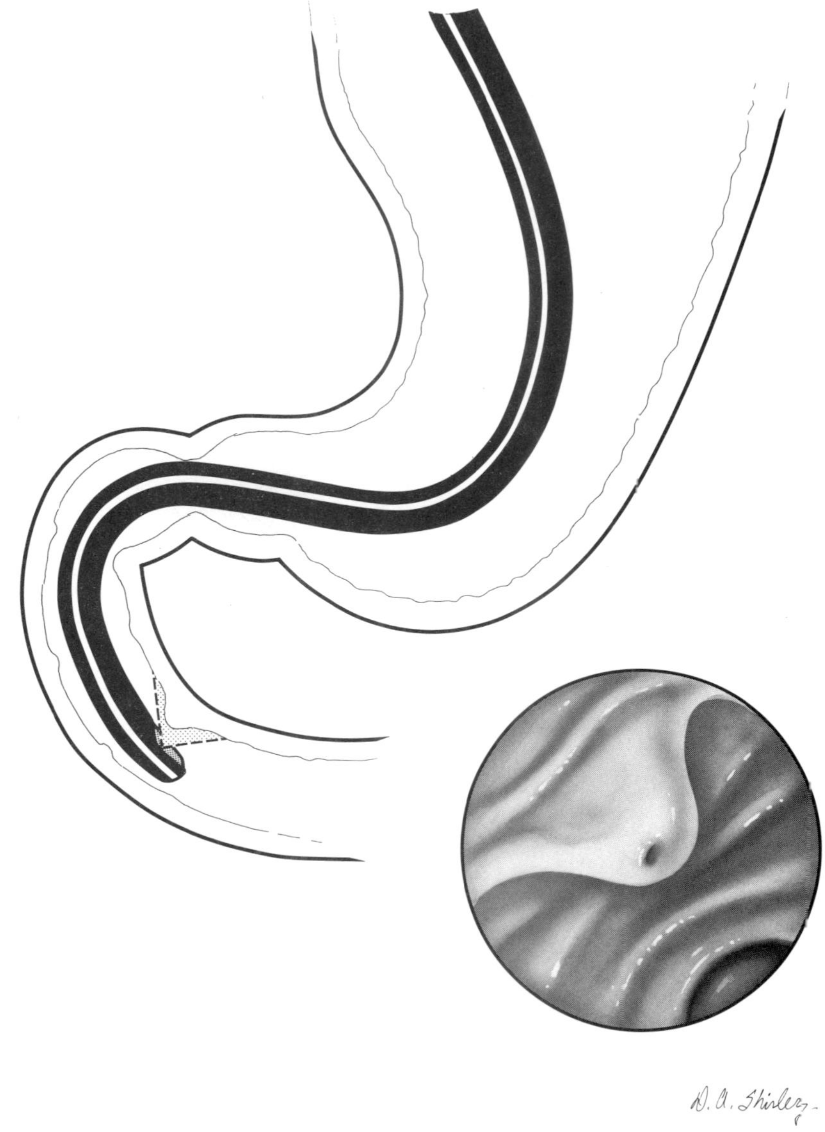

PLATE 9–6

To best approach the ampulla, the scope is straightened by elevating its tip and pulling back on its shaft. This reduces the amount of scope in the patient and causes it to lie along the lesser curvature of the stomach. This position typically brings the ampulla close to the viewing lens and in optimal position for cannulation. It is particularly useful in cannulation and manipulation of the bile duct, while the long-scope configuration may occasionally be more advantageous in approaching the pancreatic duct.

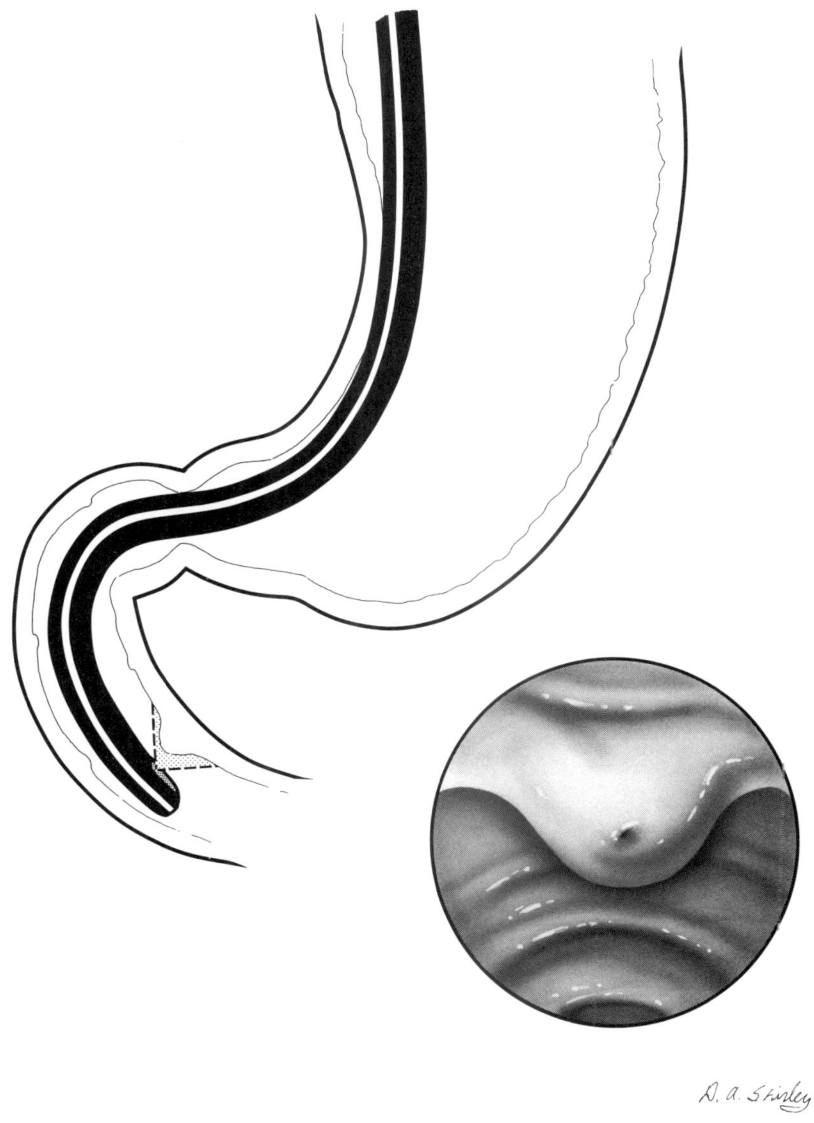

PLATE 9–7

Once an *en face* view of the ampulla is achieved, careful inspection of its surface is performed. A soft, reticulated area marks its orifice. A cannula, preflushed with contrast, is passed through the instrument channel and directed into the ampullary orifice with the aid of an elevator control on the scope. This elevator permits the endoscopist to make fine adjustments in the course of the cannula. Care should be taken to avoid excessive trauma to the ampulla, as trauma may make cannulation difficult. The bile duct courses within the duodenal wall for a short distance above the ampulla and therefore is best approached tangentially. Its orifice within the ampulla is usually superior to that of the pancreatic duct and in the 11 o'clock position. The pancreatic duct exits the ampulla perpendicularly and its orifice is usually in the 1 o'clock position within the ampulla. Frequently there is a short common channel and both ducts may be filled with a single injection. Care must be taken not to overfill the pancreatic duct, as pancreatitis is a likely result. Filling of the ducts must be monitored fluoroscopically and must be terminated when ductal filling is complete. One must avoid extravasation of contrast into the pancreatic substance (acinarization).

The variations in biliary anatomy are familiar to the surgeon, who encounters them frequently during transhepatic and operative cholangiography. The biliary ductal system should be completely filled. Preflushing of the cannula will help to prevent air bubbles, which may be confused with ductal calculi. Irregularities in the walls of the duct, filling defects, and strictures may indicate disease.

The details of pancreatic ductal structure may be less familiar. Normally, the pancreatic duct is widest near the ampulla of Vater and gradually tapers toward the tail of the gland. Dilation, tortuosity, stricture, or filling defects may indicate disease and warrant careful study.

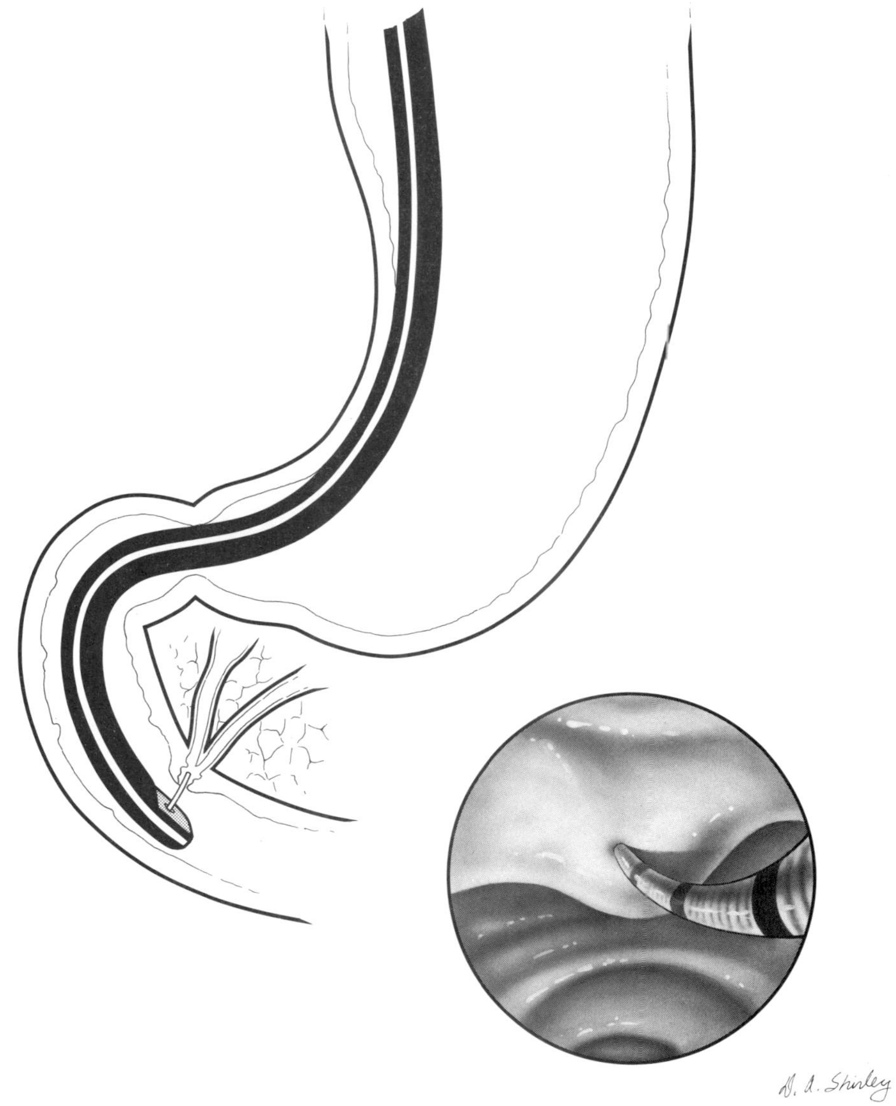

10

Endoscopic Sphincterotomy

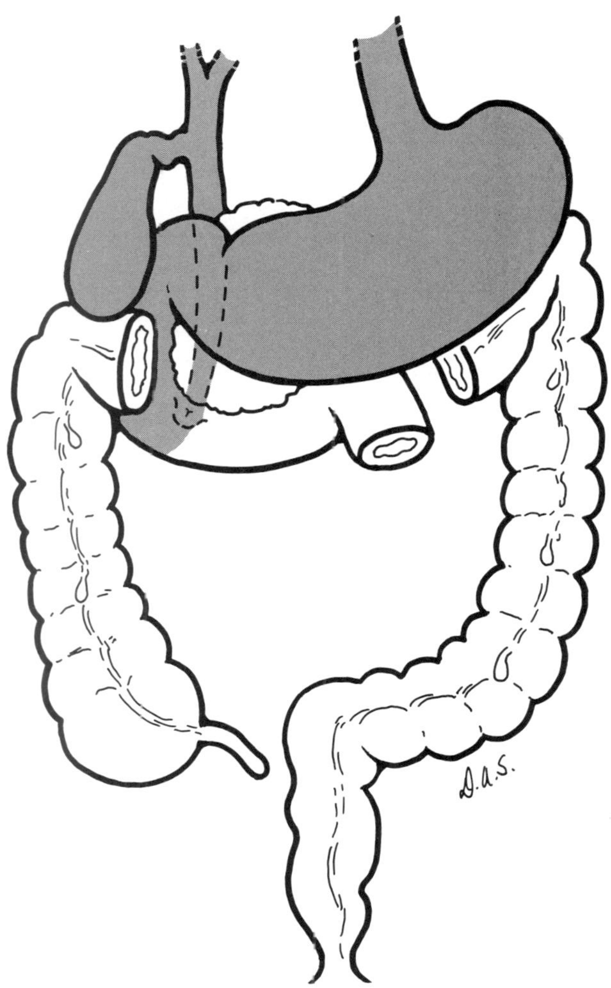

PLATE 10–1

When diagnostic ERCP reveals biliary obstruction by common bile duct calculi, the endoscopist should be prepared to perform endoscopic division of the ampullary sphincter. Other indications may include ampullary stenosis, ampullary dyskinesia, tumors of the ampulla, and the need for ductal access for endoscopic therapy in the more proximal biliary tree. Common bile duct stones are by far the most frequent indication for this procedure.

When preoperative assessment suggests the presence of stones it is often useful to perform ERCP using a double-channel sphincterotome cannula. One channel permits injection of contrast medium into the bile duct, while the other carries a cutting wire to be used for division of the sphincter. Once selective cannulation has been documented by injection of contrast medium and if sphincterotomy is deemed appropriate, the cannula is in good position to begin sectioning of the sphincter **(A).** Division of the ampulla is performed in a stepwise manner using a combination of cutting and coagulation current. The wire of the sphincterotome should be positioned so that it lies in the 11 to 12 o'clock position of the papilla. If cutting is performed in the 1 o'clock or 2 o'clock position, hemorrhage and pancreatitis are more likely. If the procedure is correctly performed, an advancing line of mucosal desiccation will appear, followed by tissue separation. The risk of hemorrhage and perforation becomes greater as the opening is made progressively larger and care should be taken not to extend the incision beyond the intramural portion of the bile duct that clearly protrudes into the duodenal lumen.

A

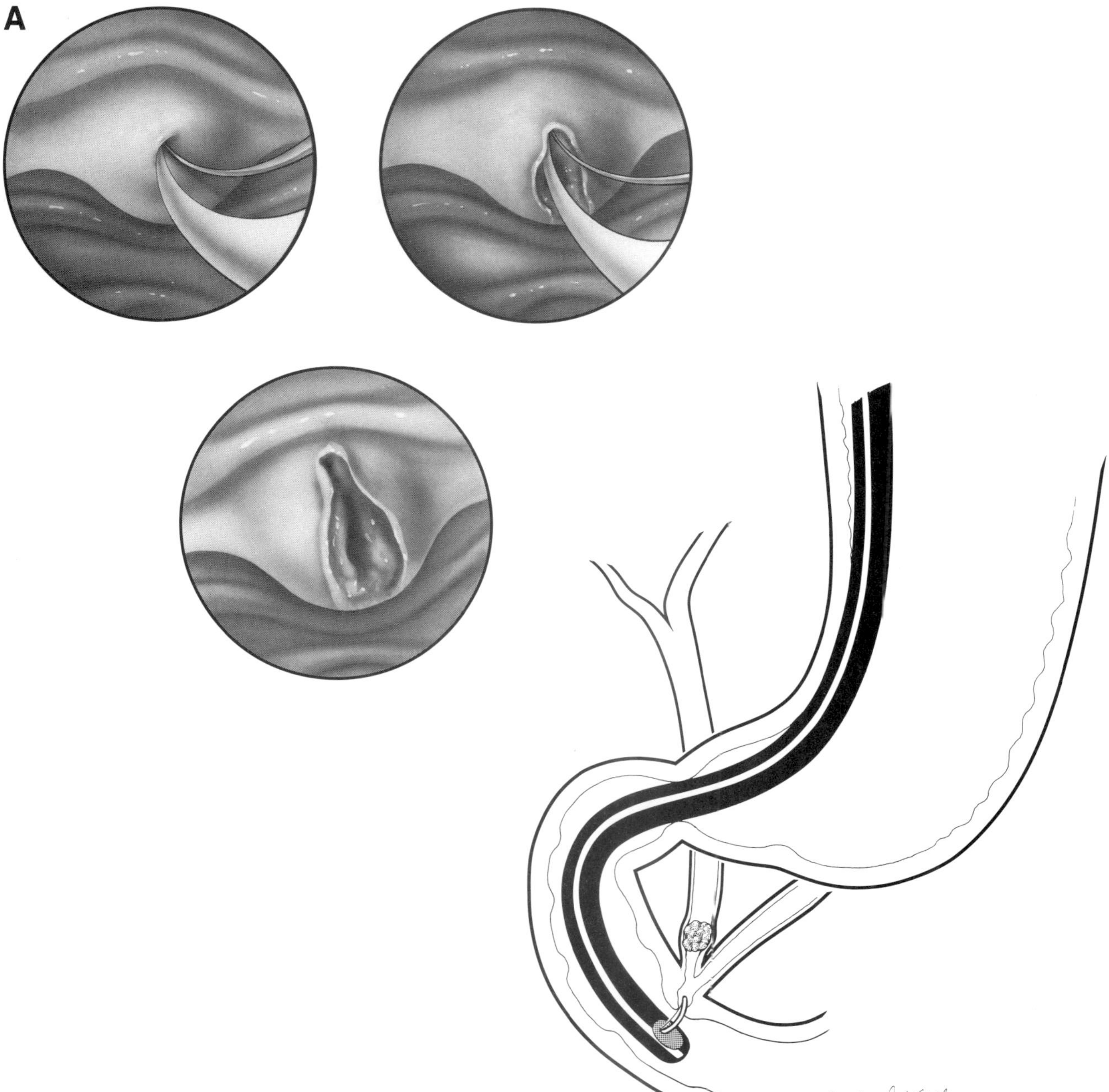

This enlarged view demonstrates the correct position of the sphincterotome as the sphincterotomy is begun **(B).** The catheter tip is selectively positioned within the common bile duct, and the endoscopist inserts only as much of the cannula as is required to cut. This may be judged by observing the black markings on the cannula, which are 3 mm apart, and prevents a massive incision from being unintentionally made should precipitous tissue separation occur. As the tissue separates, the sphincterotome can be advanced into the duct until the sphincterotomy is of desired length.

B

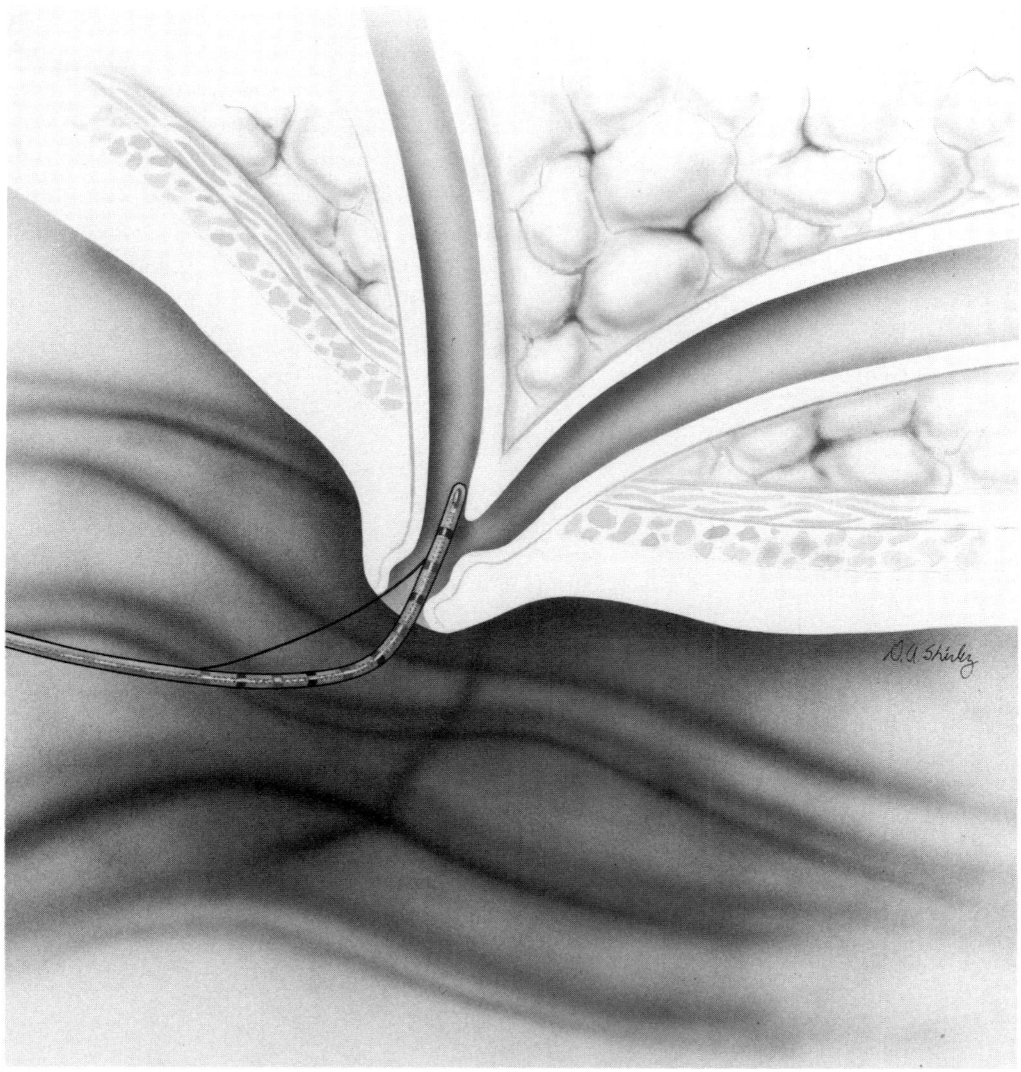

PLATE 10–2

Occasionally, as in ampullary stenosis, free cannulation cannot be achieved. In such instances, an ERCP may be obtained by impacting the cannula against the mouth of the papilla. When sphincterotomy is indicated, it may be necessary to use a precut sphincterotome. The cutting wire exits directly from the tip of such a cannula and cutting is performed in small increments in the anticipated direction of the bile duct. Once entry into the duct is achieved, the sphincterotome is selectively passed into the duct and the incision enlarged in the usual fashion. Precut sphincterotomy is less controlled and carries greater risk than the standard method. It should only be performed by those extremely skilled in endoscopic sphincterotomy.

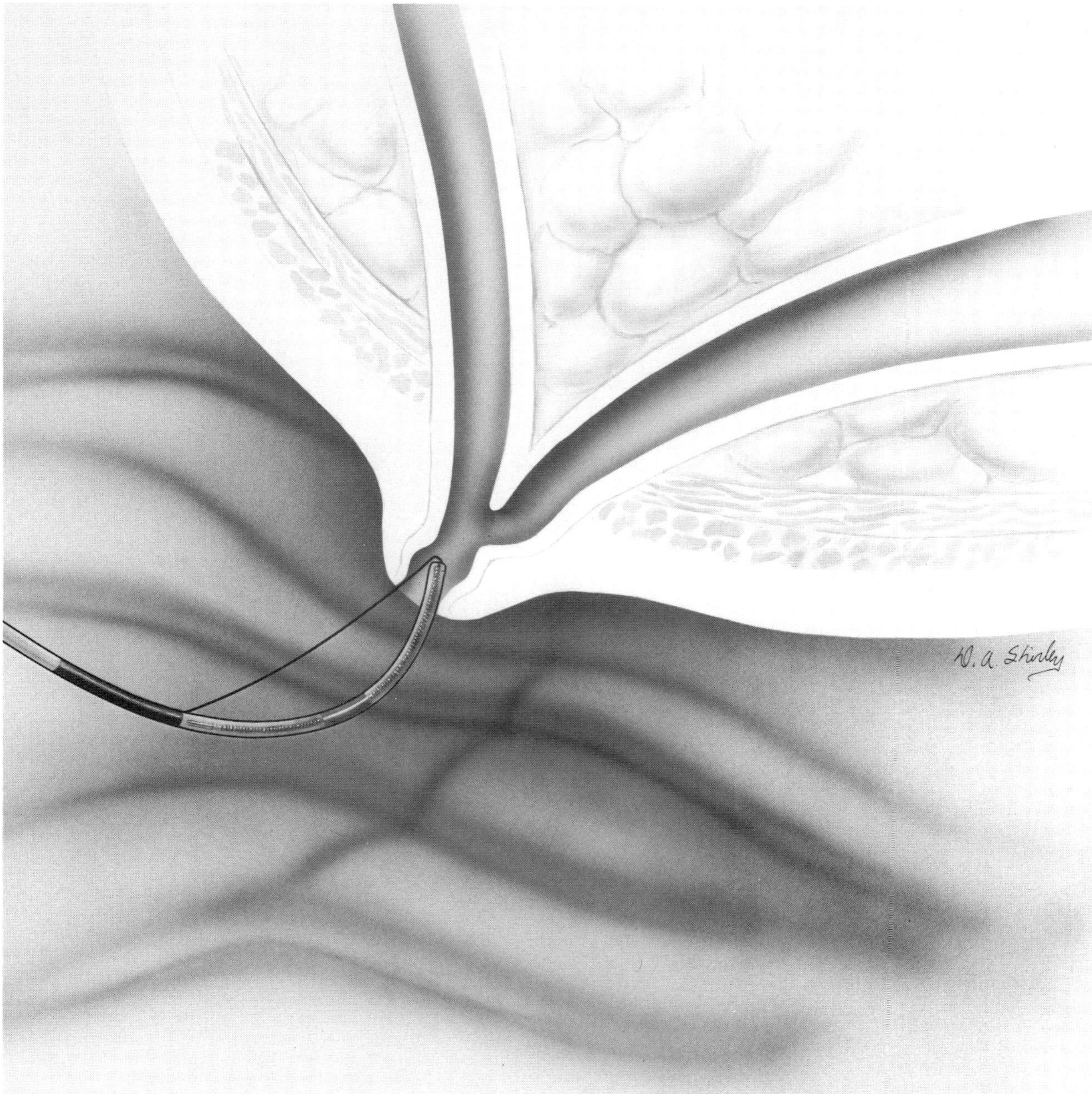

11

Extraction of Common Bile Duct Stones

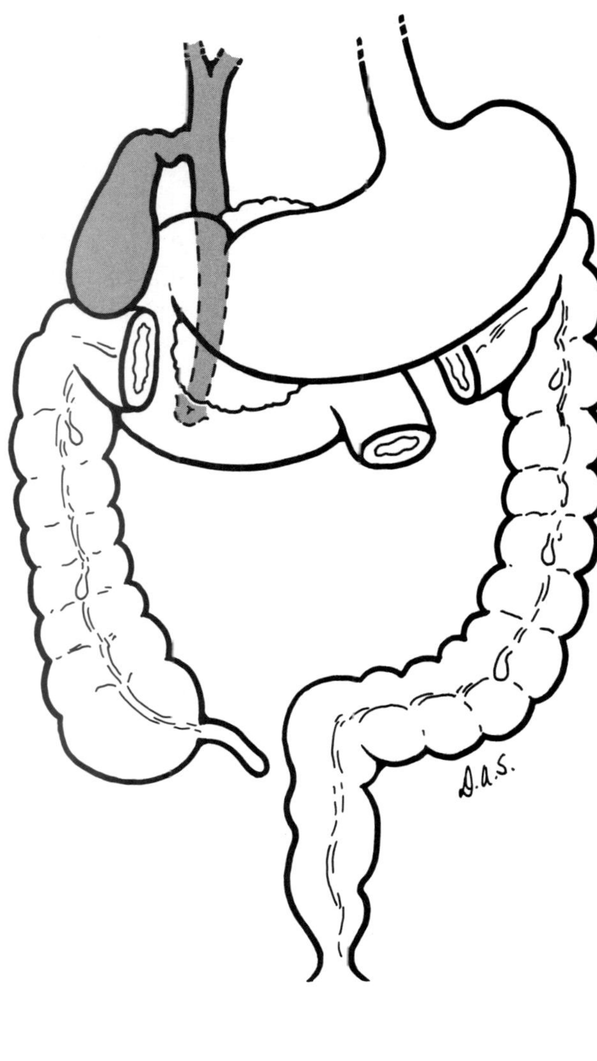

PLATE 11–1

The greatest therapeutic impact of ERCP has been the ability to identify and remove stones from the common bile duct. Choledocholithiasis following previous cholecystectomy is the most frequent indication for this intervention, but it is also appropriately applied to relieve obstruction in patients with intact gallbladders deemed unfit to undergo surgery, in the relief of acute gallstone pancreatitis, and more recently, in removing common duct stones prior to planned laparoscopic cholecystectomy.

In patients with suspected choledocholithiasis, a preliminary diagnostic ERCP must first be performed to ascertain that stones are actually present. Either a routine ERCP cannula or a double-channel sphincterotome may be used to perform the examination employed. The advantage of the latter is that contrast medium may be injected selectively into the bile duct after cannulation. Should stones be identified, the wire will be in good position to perform the sphincterotomy incision, avoiding the need for recannulation. Tiny stones may occasionally be flushed from the duct without sphincterotomy. Removal of most stones, however, will require division of the sphincter. The size of the sphincterotomy will be predicated upon the largest diameter of the stone to be removed and the length of intramural bile duct visible in the duodenal wall. Since the sphincterotomy carries more risk of bleeding and perforation as it is extended, it should be no longer than required for stone extraction and should not be carried beyond the visible intramural portion of the bile duct. Cannulation of the bile duct and manipulation of stones are usually best carried out with the duodenoscope in the lesser-curvature or short-scope configuration.

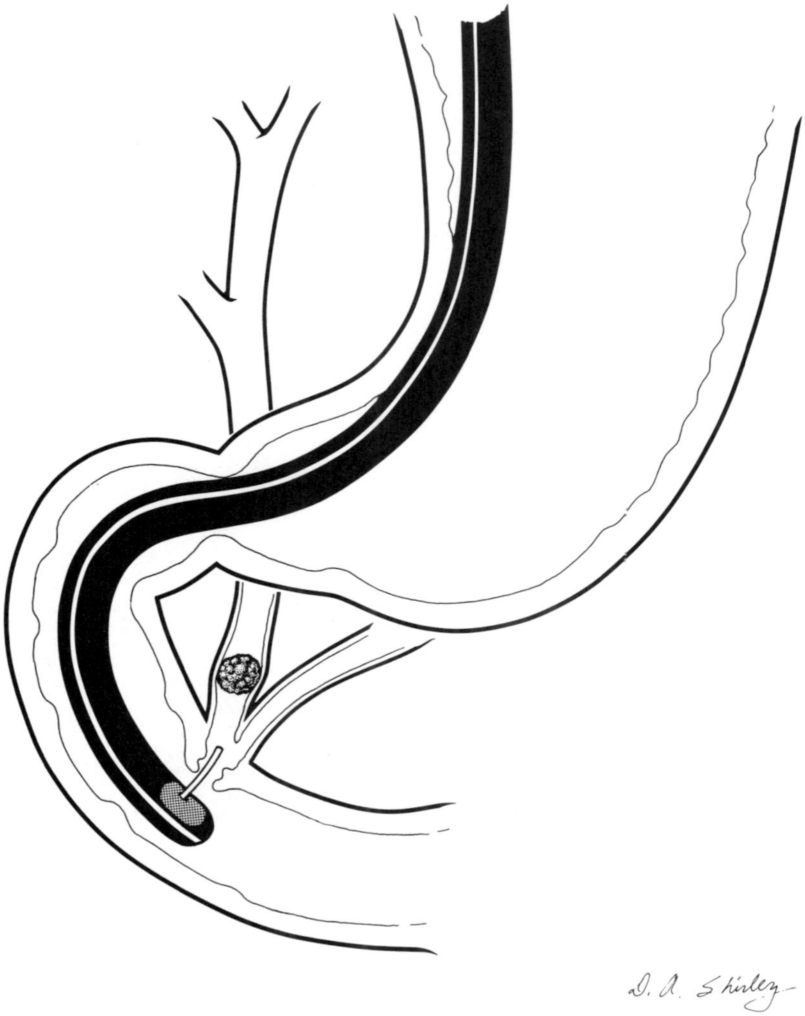

PLATE 11–2

Some stones will pass spontaneously immediately after division of the sphincter; others will pass within hours to days, even without further manipulation. Most endoscopists prefer to extract stones if after sphincterotomy they do not immediately pass and there is no difficulty encountered with the sphincterotomy. A balloon-tip catheter, usually inflatable to 15 mm, is introduced into the duct and manipulated so that its tip is proximal to the most distal stone. The balloon is inflated with air and gently pulled downward with steady traction to coax the stone through the open sphincter. This technique is quite safe and effective.

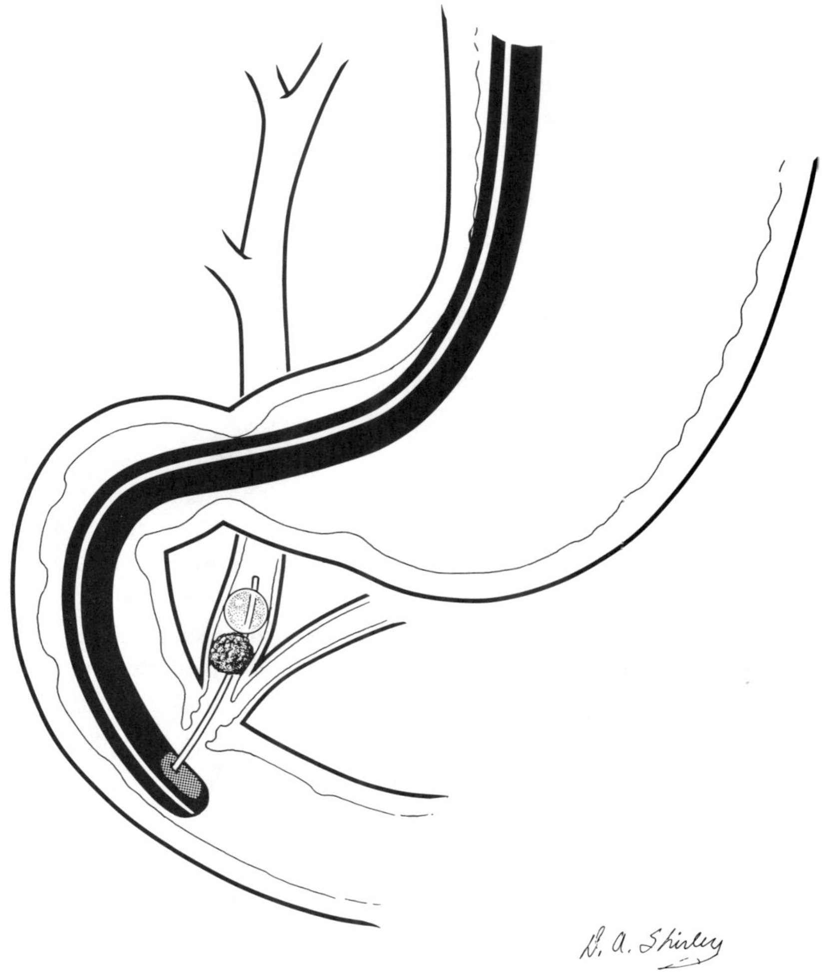

PLATE 11–3

Stones that seem unsuited to balloon extraction may be approached by use of a wire basket **(A).** The closed basket is advanced into the duct proximal to the most distal stone. The basket is then opened and the catheter pulled backward so that the basket lies in the area of the stone. It is usually necessary to "jiggle" the basket back and forth next to the stone until the stone moves into the arms of the basket.

Once the stone is within the basket, the basket may be closed a bit and slowly withdrawn from the duct **(B).** Some endoscopists prefer to withdraw the basket without closing it, fearing that the stone may be prematurely crushed or lost by closing the basket. If basket attempts at stone removal are successful, additional passes of the basket are made. Each time, the most distal remaining stone is addressed and removed.

Should the stone be surrounded and be refractory to removal through the sphincterotomy, several options exist. The endoscopist may choose to open the basket and try to release the stone. This failing, the basket wire may be cut at the operator's end of the scope. The scope may be removed, leaving the basket in place. Then a metal sheath can be threaded over the basket wire and a lithotripsy device attached that will force the metal sheath against the basket and crush the stone (or break the basket). Alternatively, the initial basket used may be one designed for lithotripsy. Should the stone not be easily extractable, the basket may be tightened firmly and the stone crushed without the need to remove the endoscope. The latter type of basket is the one of choice and will be most widely used in the future. Such crushing of the stone with a basket is termed *mechanical lithotripsy*.

When basket removal of the stone or stone fragments is accomplished, the stone or debris is pulled into the duodenal lumen and released **(C).** It is not necessary to remove these stones from the intestine as they rarely are of a size that would produce distal obstruction.

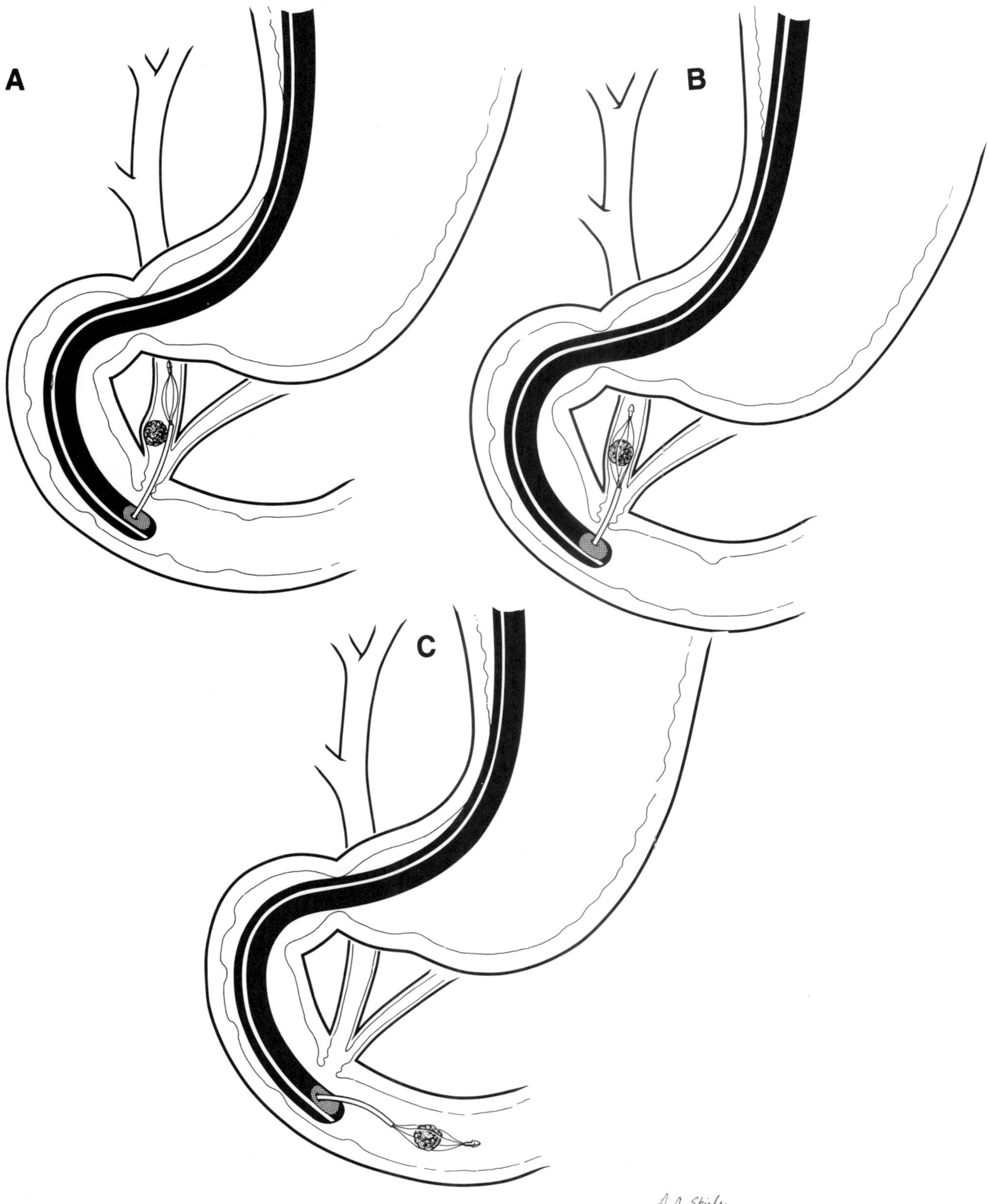
A
B
C

PLATE 11–4

Electrohydraulic lithotripsy devices are available that transmit a powerful pulse of energy to a stone in order to shatter it. These bipolar electrical devices must be applied directly to the surface of the stone. The wall of the common duct may be injured if the energy is misdirected. Special balloon catheters are available through which the lithotripsy electrode may be passed in order to prevent the electrode from touching the bile duct walls.

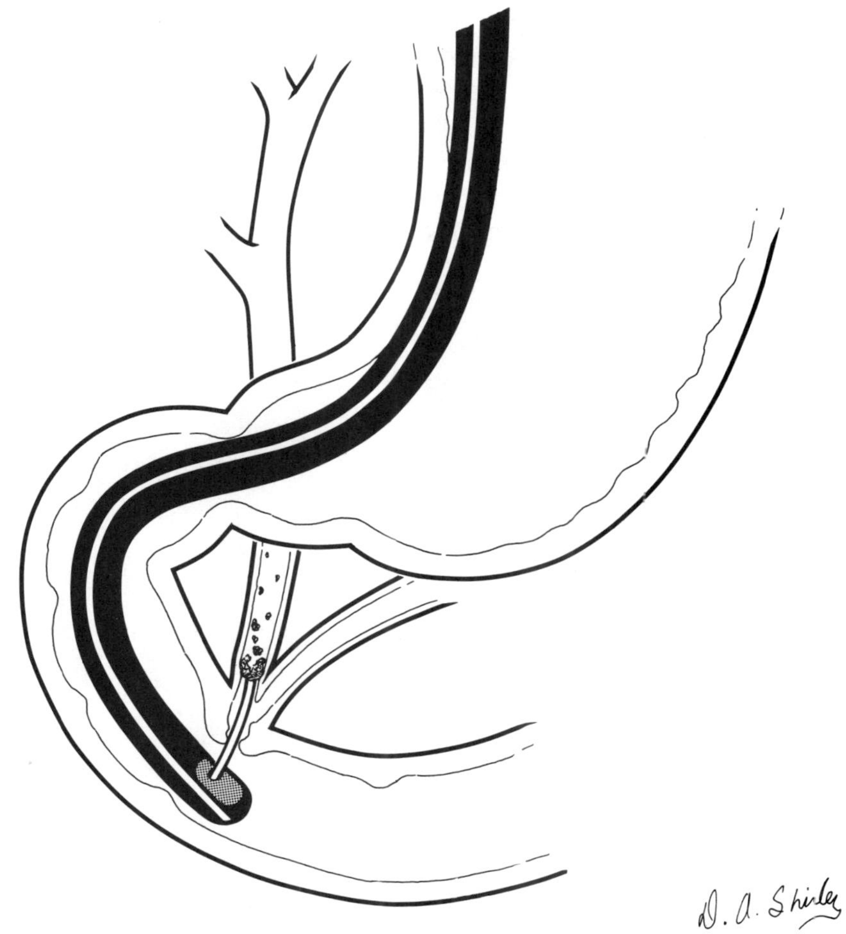

PLATE 11–5

Difficult or very large stones may be approached using a "mother-daughter" endoscope system. The "mother" scope replaces the standard duodenoscope and the "daughter" instrument is passed through the lumen of the larger. A generous sphincterotomy must be available for passage of the instrument and its passage requires skilled manipulation. Once within the common duct, the daughter scope may be used to visualize the stone and manipulate it. Laser lithotripsy may be employed through the biopsy channel of the daughter scope. The most effective laser for such therapy is the pulse dye laser. Here, too, the laser must be in direct contact with the stone to be effective; however, this type of laser produces minimal damage to the bile duct.

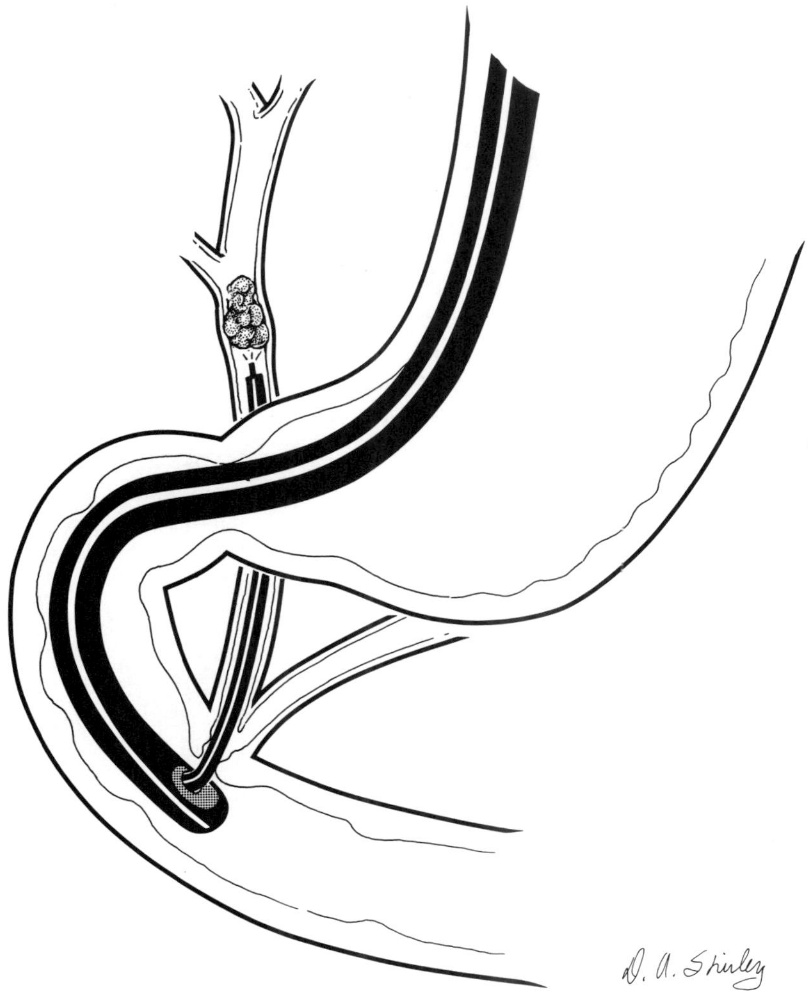
D. A. Shirley

PLATE 11–6

Following extraction of what is believed to be the last stone, a completion cholangiogram should be obtained to document that there are no further stones within the duct. Small fragments that may be seen within the duct, but which will clearly pass through the wide sphincterotomy, may occasionally be left to pass spontaneously.

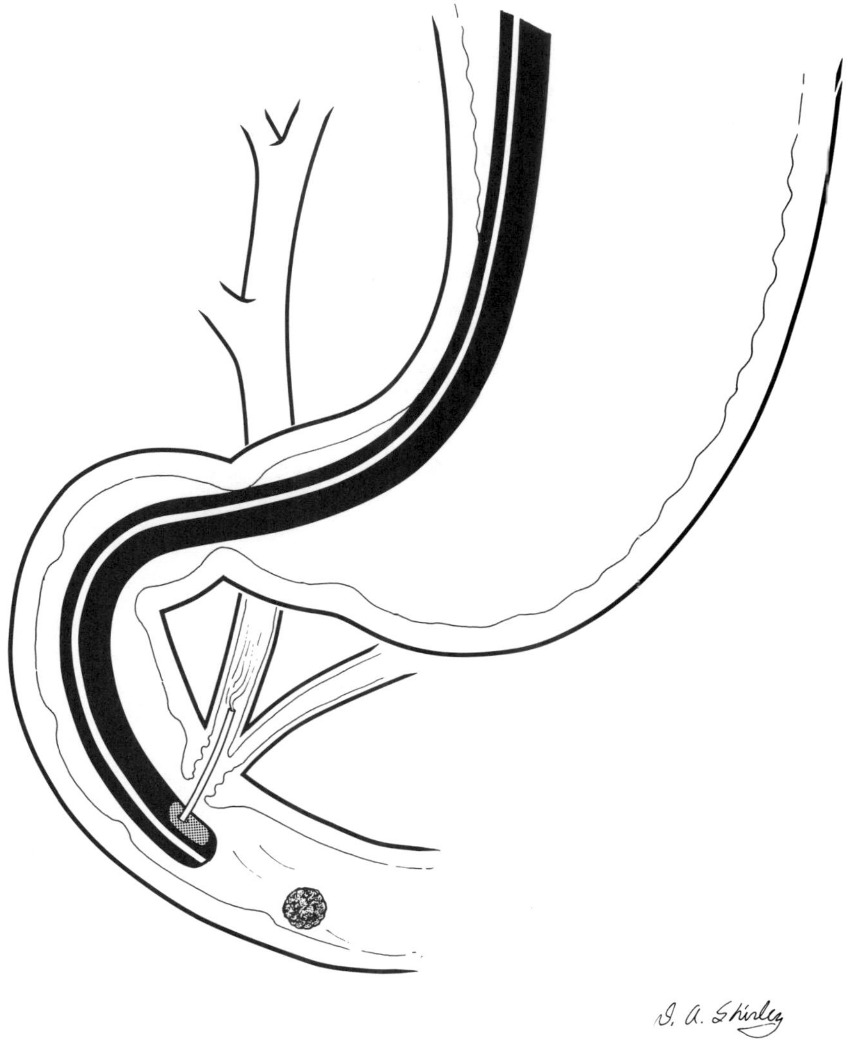

PLATE 11–7

At times, very large or multiple stones may preclude safe or complete clearance of the common bile duct by endoscopic means. In some cases this will dictate the need for surgical exploration; however, in very aged or infirm patients, satisfactory drainage may be achieved by use of a nasobiliary drain or stent placed into the duct above the stones. The drain will require replacement at intervals, but may provide an attractive alternative to surgery.

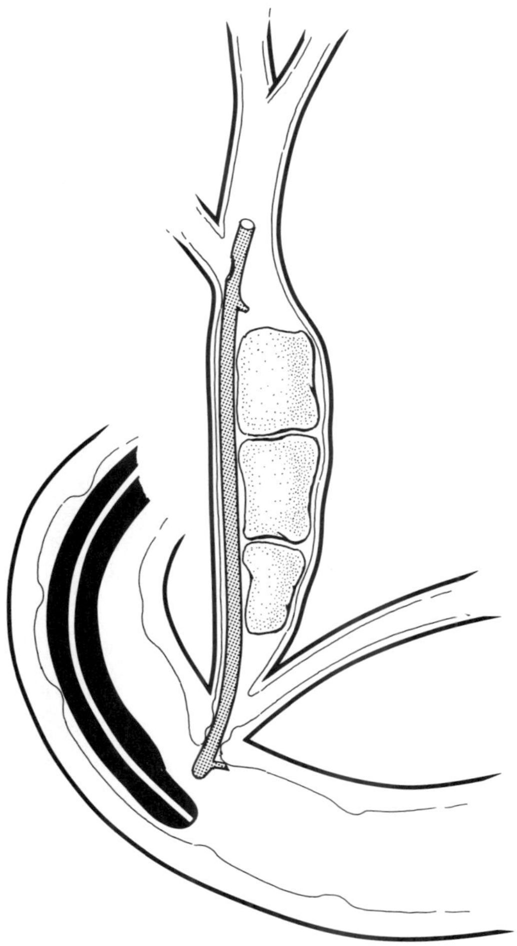

PLATE 11–8

Some authors have reported chemical dissolution of gallbladder stones by means of endoscopic retrograde cystic duct cannulation. In these cases, a long naso-cholecystic tube is passed via the ampulla through the cystic duct and into the gallbladder. Chemical agents such as mono-octanoin or methyl tertiary butyl ether may be infused to dissolve cholesterol gallstones. This method remains investigational.

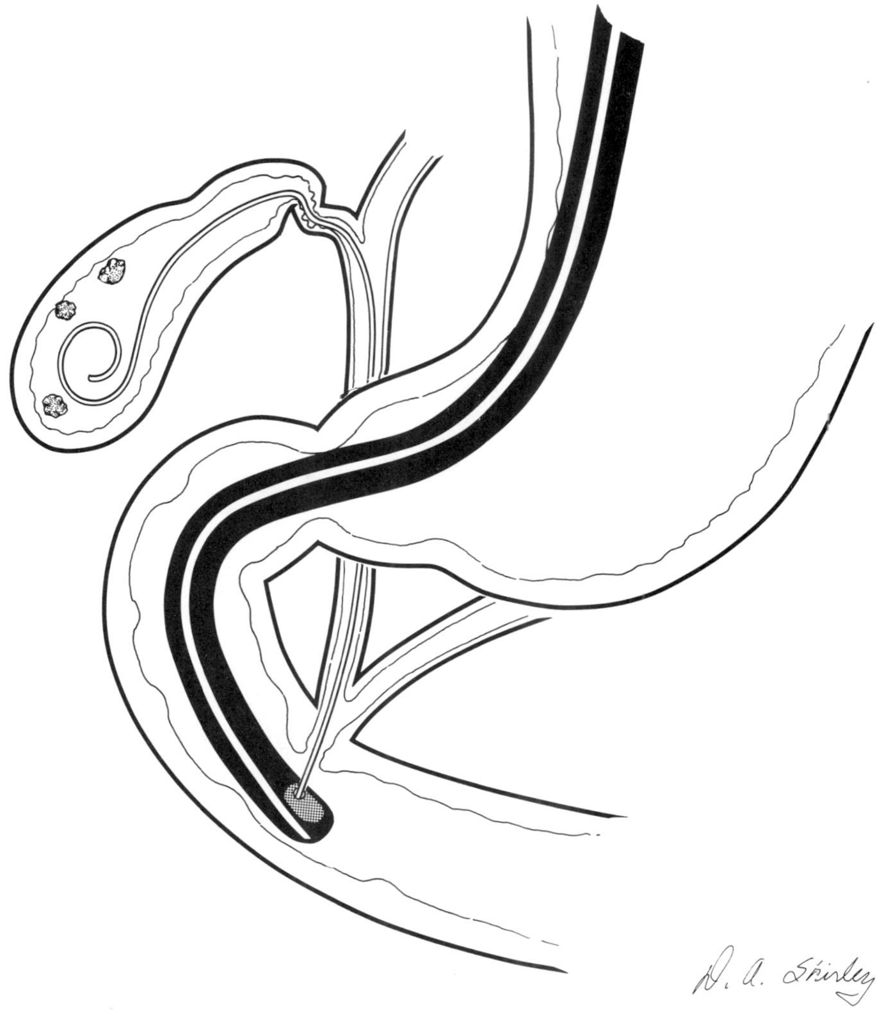
D. A. Shirley

12

Dilation of Bile Duct Strictures

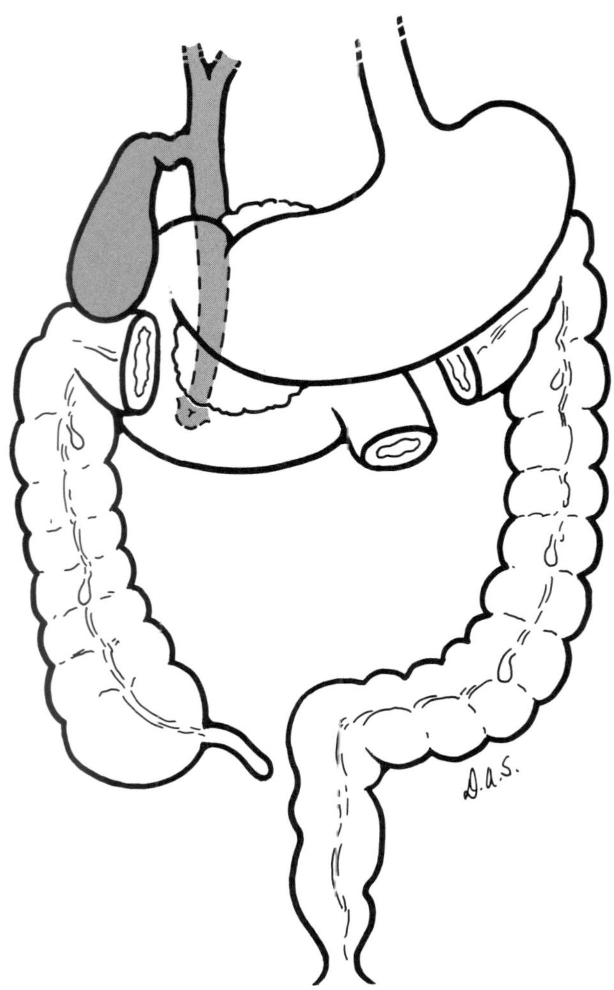

PLATE 12–1

Strictures of the bile ducts may be the result of benign disease, iatrogenic injury, malignant neoplasm, pancreatitis, extrinsic compression, ischemic injury, or sclerosing cholangitis. In general, strictures of the duct are difficult to dilate and after opening frequently revert to their narrowed state; however, dilation may be appropriate as initial therapy and prior to stenting.

This schematic drawing demonstrates a focal stricture near the junction of the cystic duct stump. Such strictures can occur following injury to the bile duct during cholecystectomy. A careful diagnostic ERCP must first be performed to evaluate the length and degree of narrowing.

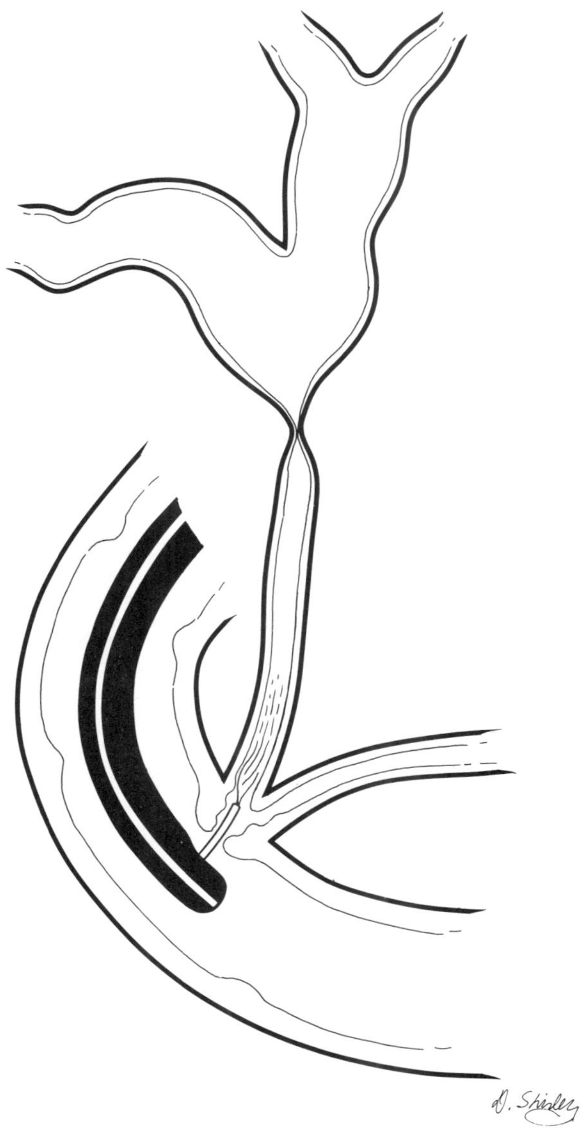

PLATE 12–2

A firm dilating balloon of the desired caliber and length can be passed through the stricture. In some cases it may be necessary to first pass a wire, then pass the balloon over the wire through the area of narrowing **(A).**

Under fluoroscopic guidance, the balloon is inflated with contrast agent. This is done slowly, so as not to cause tearing and to allow gradual stretching of the tissue. A pressure gauge is used so as not to exceed the maximum inflation pressure for the balloon. Initially, a narrowed area (or waist) will appear at the central portion of the balloon, indicating the area of the stricture **(B).**

With gradual and steady inflation, dilation should proceed until the waist of the balloon no longer is seen fluoroscopically, indicating the balloon has been dilated to its full diameter **(C).** Inflation is maintained for several minutes. The balloon is then deflated and removed from the duct. Several sequential dilations may be necessary.

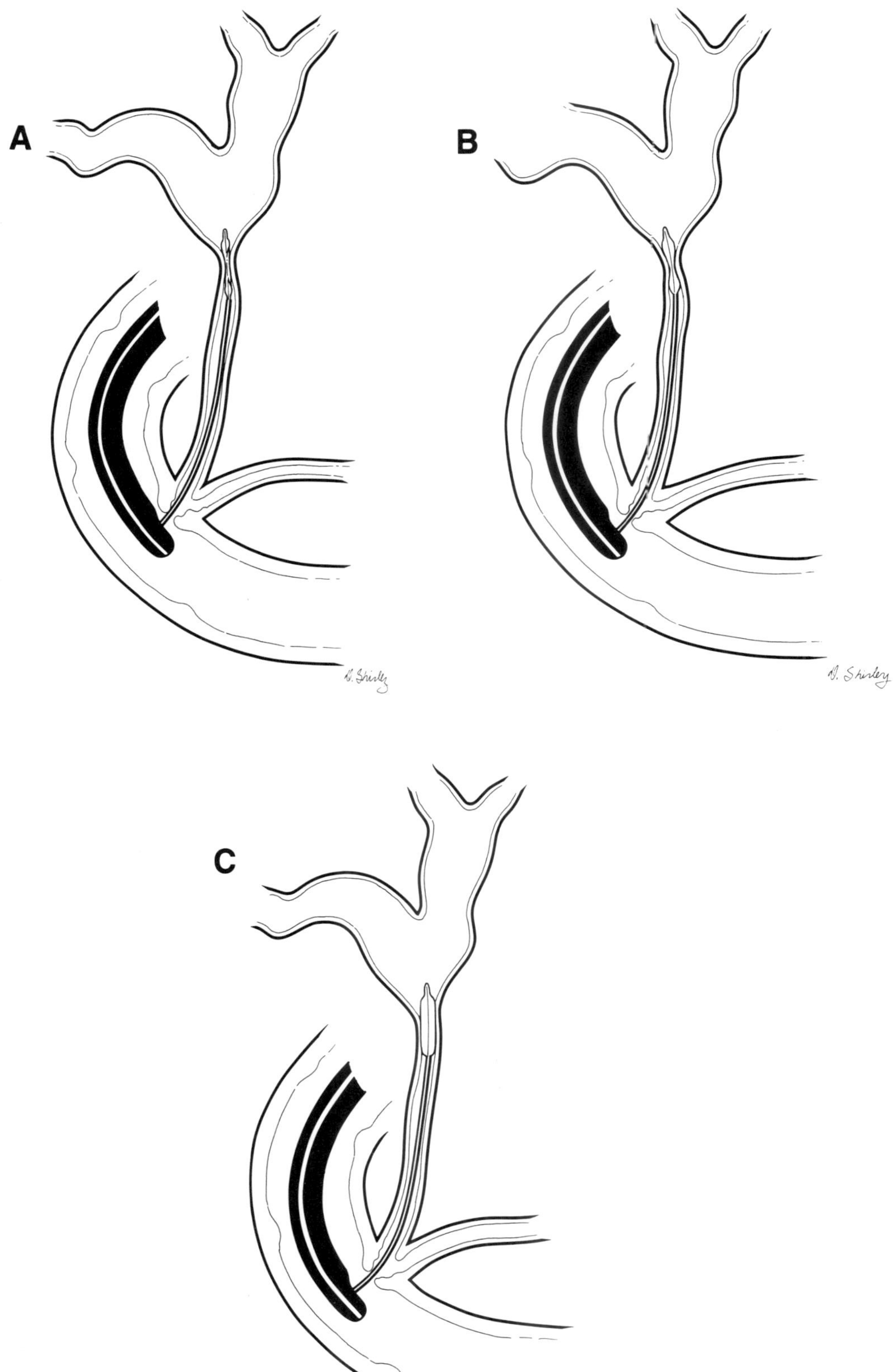
A
B
C

PLATE 12–3

A completion cholangiogram should be obtained to document the results of dilation and ascertain whether further immediate therapy is warranted.

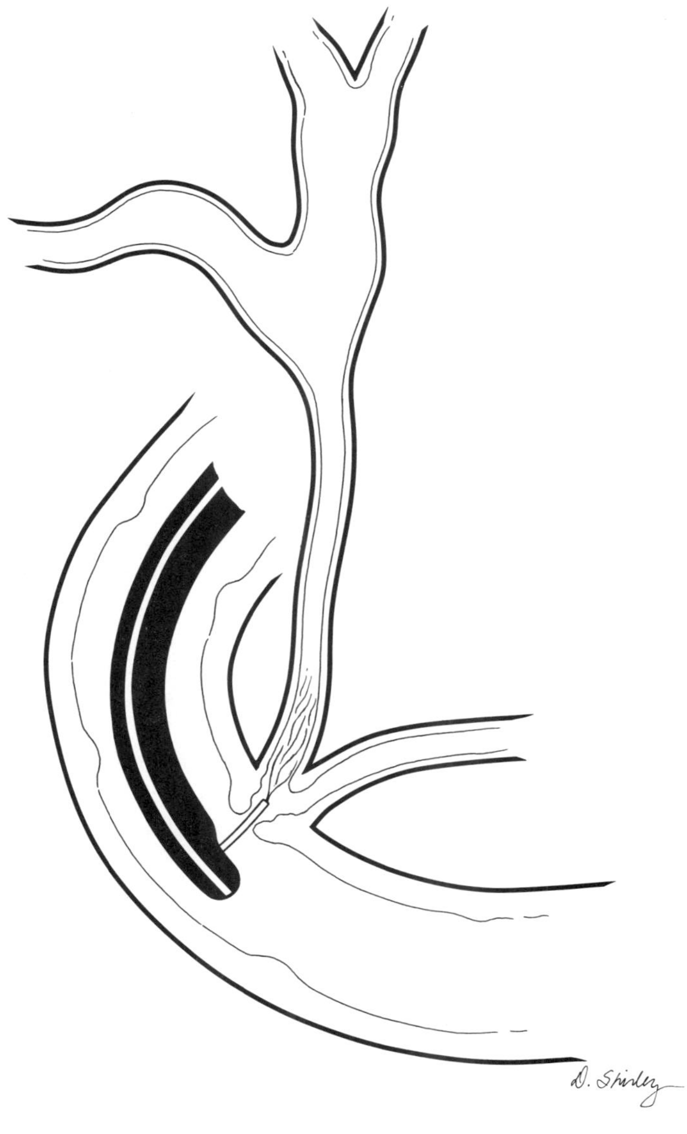

13

Endoscopic Placement of Bile Duct Stents

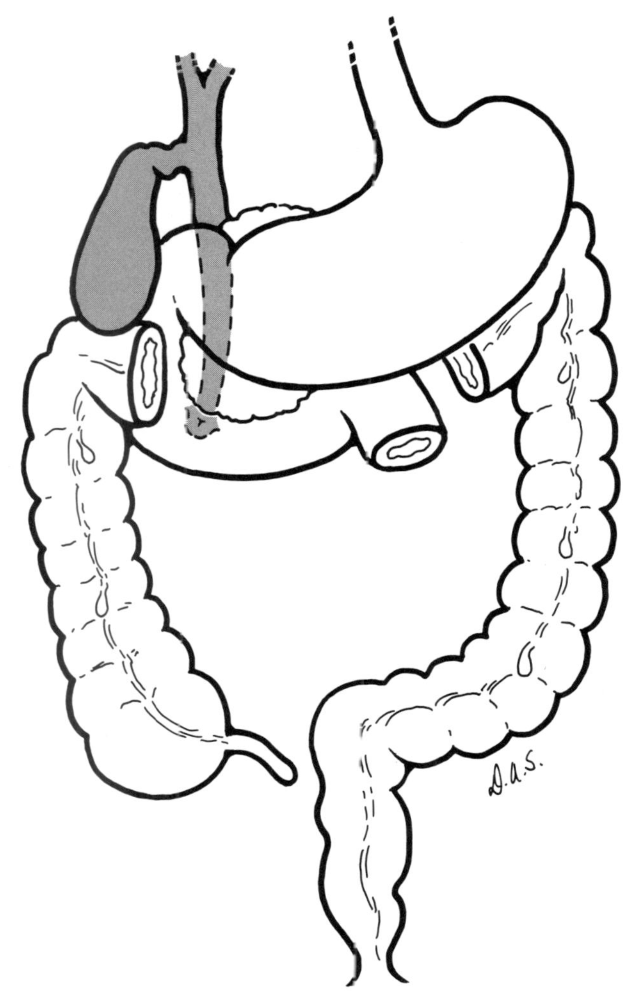

PLATE 13–1

Endoscopic placement of bile duct stents has proven useful in the palliation of unresectable malignancies of the pancreas and bile duct, in cases of extrinsic malignant obstruction of the duct, and in occasional benign conditions where surgical intervention is deemed inappropriate. Stenting is now being used in selected cases of pancreatic duct obstruction as well. A variety of stent materials and configurations are in use, but the basic method of placement is fairly standard.

A diagnostic ERCP demonstrates a double duct sign: both the bile duct and pancreatic duct are narrowed close to their duodenal junction, indicating the presence of carcinoma of the head of the pancreas. This condition is rarely curable and in most cases endoscopic stenting of the common bile duct provides biliary decompression without the need for laparotomy. In order to place stents of reasonable size (10 F or larger), the standard duodenoscope must be replaced with the larger channel instrument.

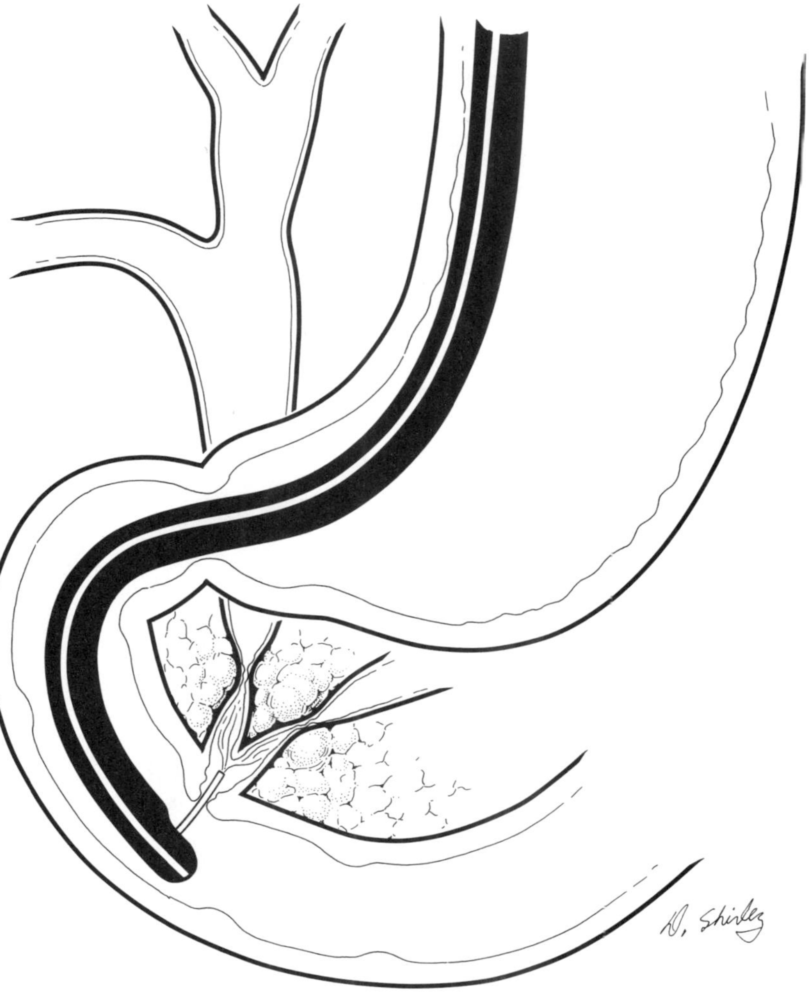
D. Shirley

PLATE 13–2

In some cases, a cannula and stent may be placed without the need for sphincterotomy; however, in most cases, a small sphincterotomy is helpful in allowing placement. If the narrowing is severe, a guide wire alone may be advanced through it into the proximal bile duct. Often the cannula covering the wire may be passed with the wire through the stricture. In difficult strictures, however, the wire itself is advanced first **(A).**

Once the wire is beyond the narrowed segment, it is passed well into the proximal bile duct and the cannula is advanced over the wire **(B).**

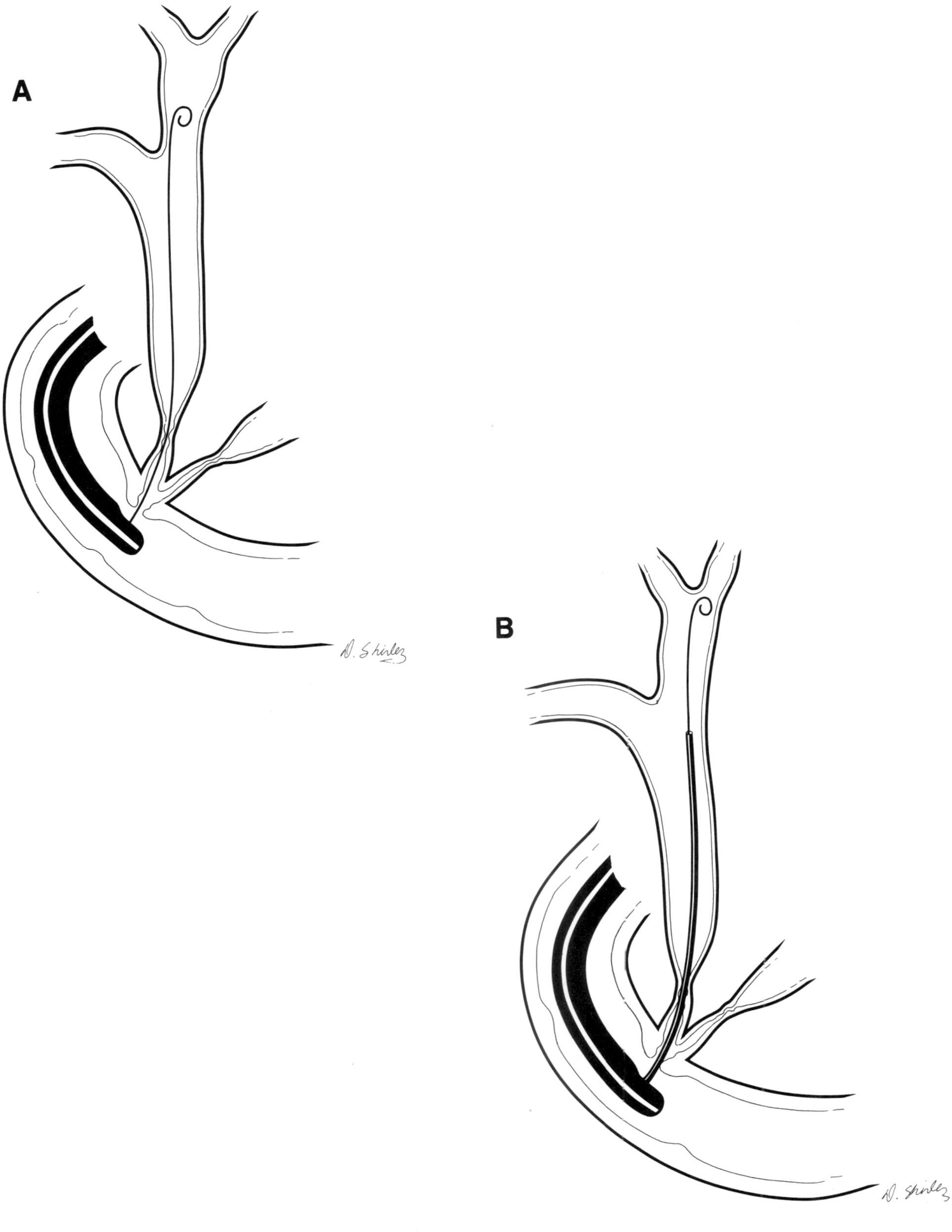
A
B

PLATE 13–3

A stent of appropriate length and caliber is selected and care is taken to assure that the stent, when in place, will extend far enough beyond the obstruction into the proximal bile duct and distally into the duodenum. The stent is passed over the cannula and a pusher tube used to move it into position. The pusher tube is a larger-caliber cannula that abuts directly against the end of the stent. The stent is advanced into the bile duct, the wire and its cannula acting as a trolley to guide it into position **(A).** Manipulation of the scope's tip toward the ampulla and upward motion of the channel elevator help to force the stent through the narrow area and into the correct position. Throughout this maneuver, the endoscopist should try to maintain a position such that the tip of the instrument is at or slightly below the ampulla so that the vector of force is in the proper direction. The tip of the instrument is best kept close to the ampulla to avoid redundancy and bowing of the stent apparatus.

When the stent is in proper position **(B),** the guide wire is removed and contrast medium may be introduced through the inner cannula to obtain a completion cholangiogram and assess drainage. The inner cannula is then removed and the scope withdrawn. The stents currently available eventually become occluded with debris and usually require replacement at 4- to 6-month intervals. Stents are easily removed by grasping them with a polypectomy snare and pulling them out. A replacement is introduced in the same manner as the first.

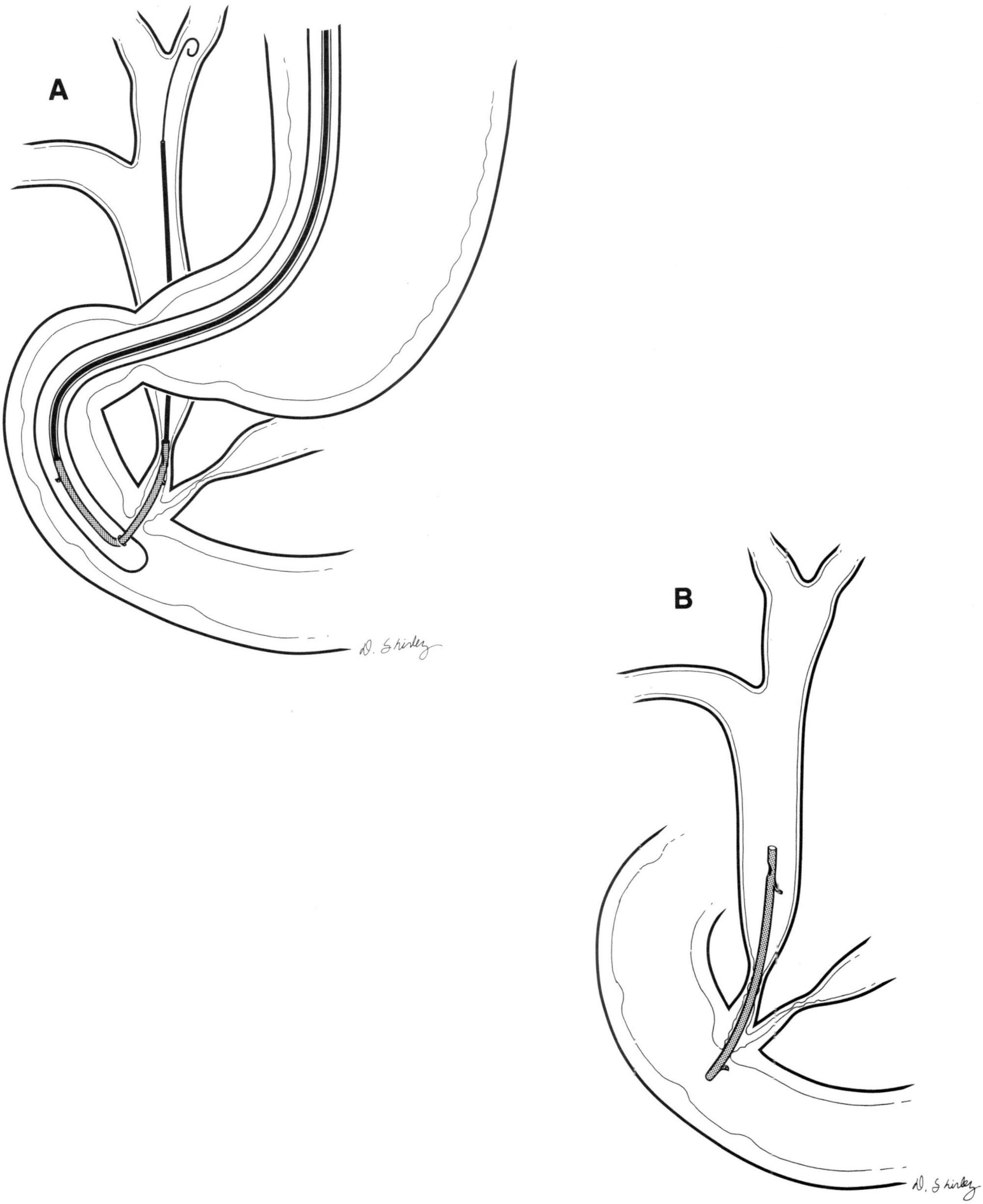
A
B

14

Endoscopic Drainage of Pancreatic Pseudocyst

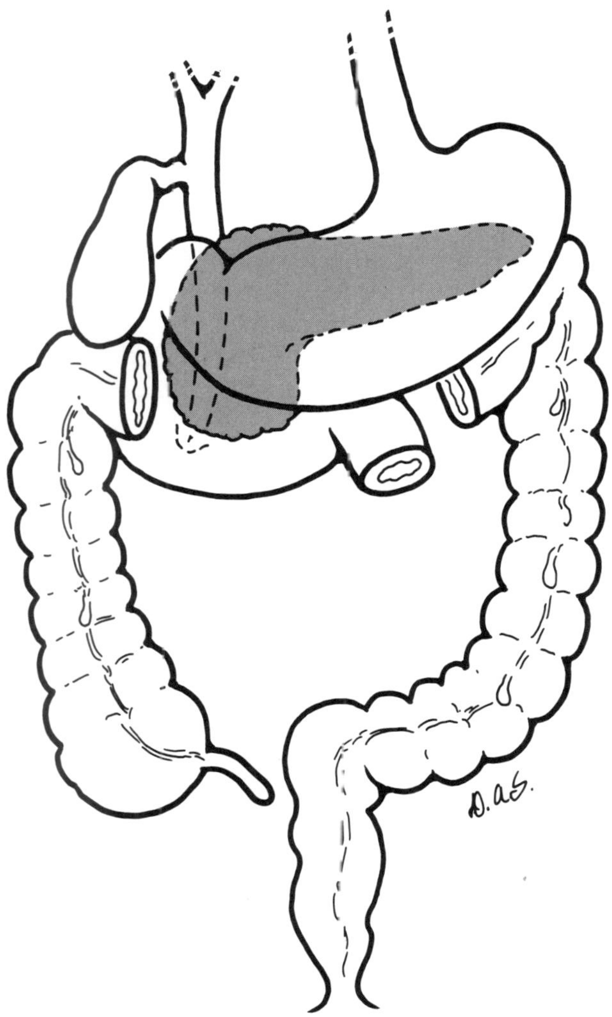

PLATE 14–1

Pancreatic pseudocysts are well-circumscribed collections of pancreatic juice outside the confines of the pancreatic ductal system. They occur as a result of ductal disruption caused by inflammation or injury. Most pseudocysts are small and many will resolve spontaneously. Computed tomographic scans are useful in following their course. Traditional surgical therapy for pseudocyst is performed after maturation of the cyst wall and involves drainage into the stomach, duodenum, or a jejunal loop. Recently, successful attempts at percutaneous and endoscopic drainage have emerged.

This figure demonstrates a pseudocyst adherent to the posterior gastric wall and protruding into the lumen of the stomach. Typically, a side-viewing duodenoscope is utilized for drainage of a pseudocyst. A needle-knife, a cutting wire in a plastic sheath, is passed through the biopsy channel of the endoscope and used to puncture the cyst with the application of a blended cutting and coagulation current. Once the puncture occurs, fluid will emerge around the catheter. The needle-knife and its sheath should be advanced well into the cavity of the cyst.

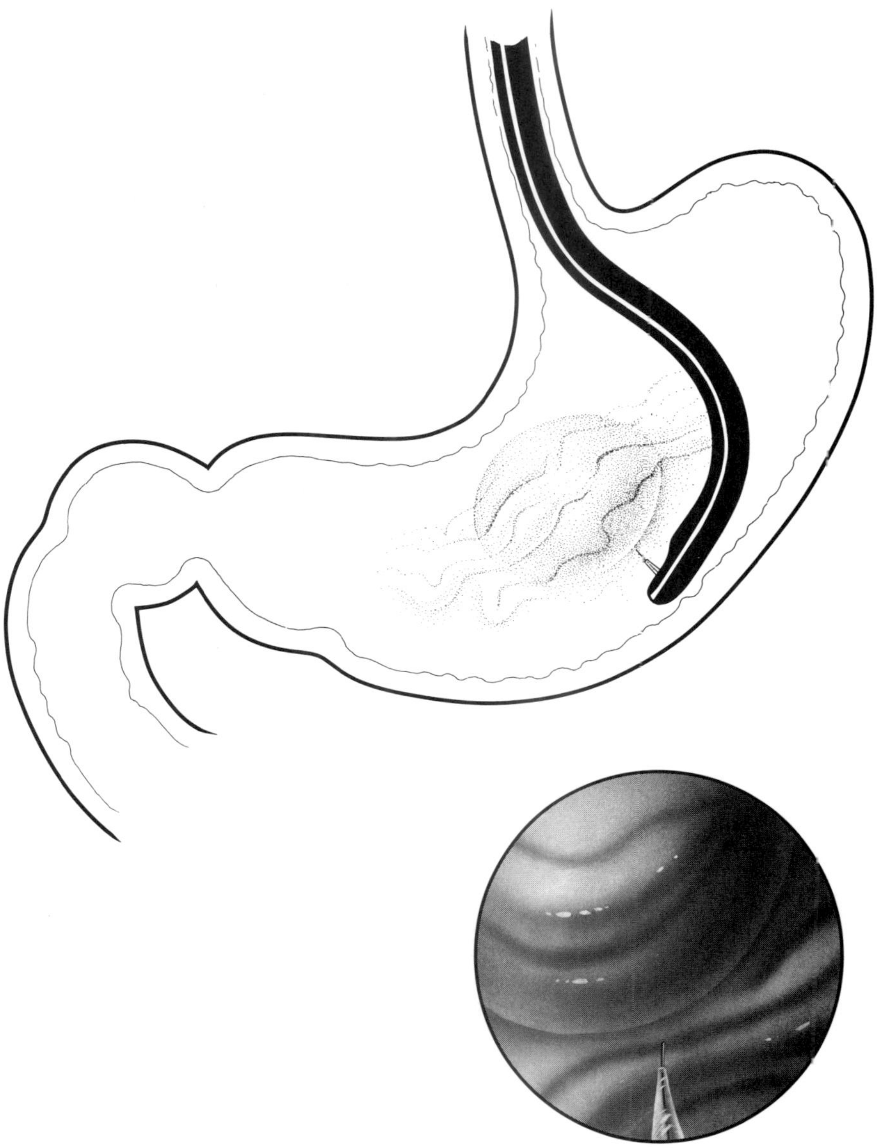

PLATE 14–2

Once the sheath is well within the cavity of the cyst, the needle is removed and replaced with a long guide wire passed through the sheath. The distal stomach is schematically removed here to better illustrate how the catheter crosses the gastric wall and enters the cyst **(A).**

The guide wire is inserted sufficiently far to curl within the cavity of the pseudocyst **(B).** The outer catheter of the needle-knife is then removed. The endoscope should be kept close to the entrance of the wire into the cyst to ensure that it does not bow in the gastric lumen.

A biliary stent is then passed over the wire and directed through the gastric wall into the cyst cavity. This is facilitated by keeping the tip of the scope close to the puncture site and using the biopsy channel elevator of the instrument to help advance the stent into the cyst **(C).**

A

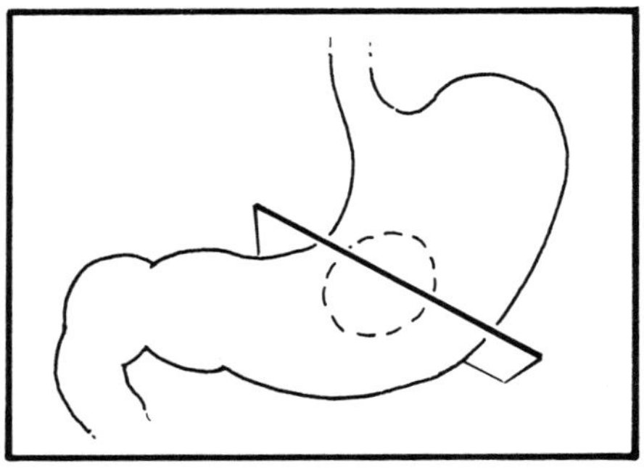

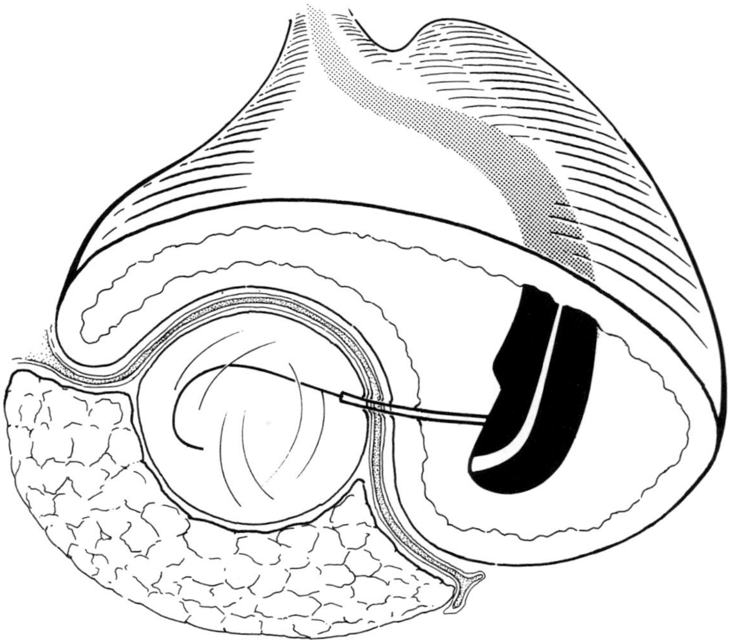

D.A.S.

B

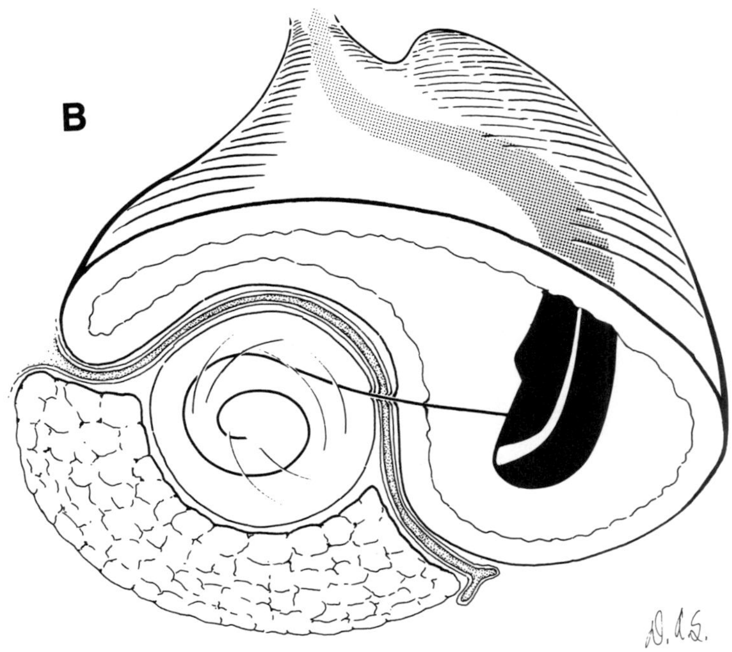

C

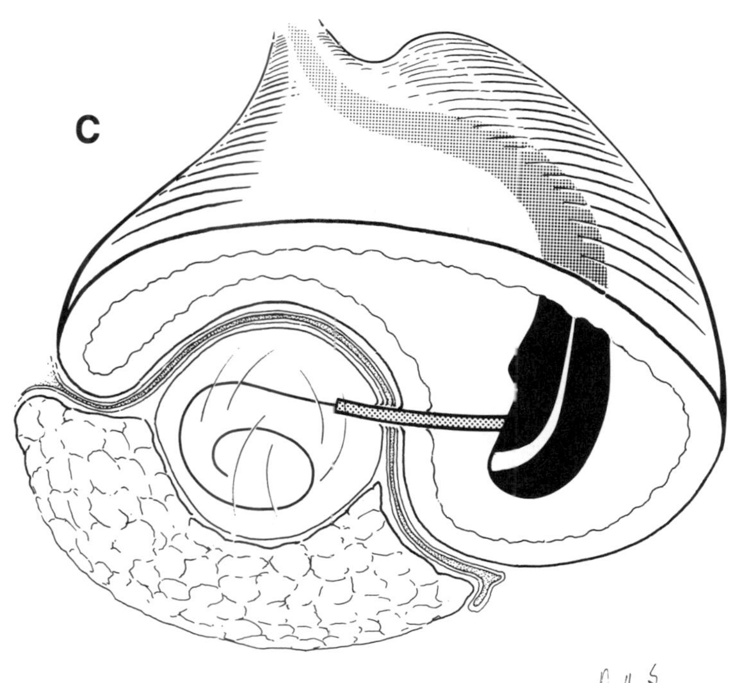

PLATE 14–3

After insertion of the stent into the cavity of the cyst, the guide wire is removed. Cyst fluid will be seen to drain into the gastric lumen and cyst decompression may be documented on CT scans. After approximately 6 weeks, with complete disappearance of the pseudocyst, the stent may be removed by securing it within a polypectomy snare and removing it with traction.

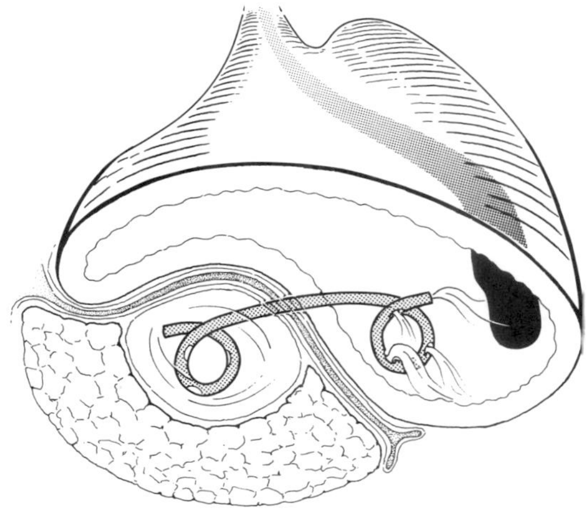

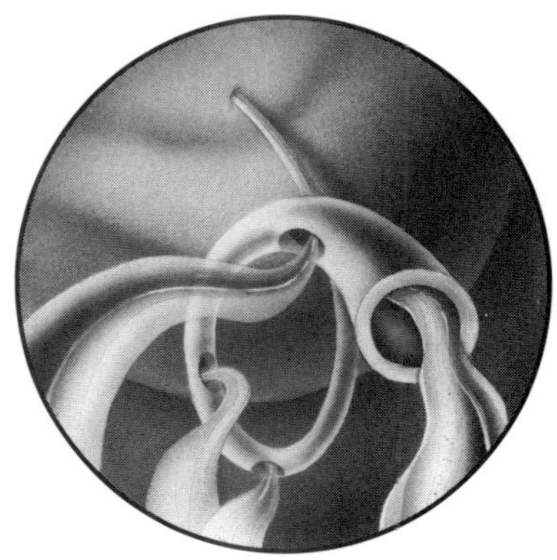

15

Choledochoscopy

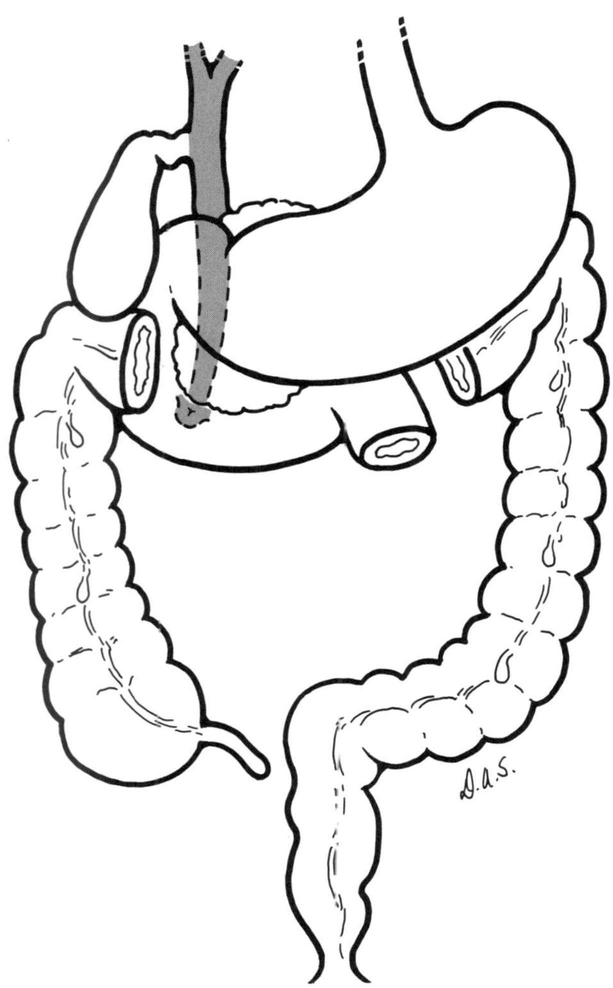

PLATE 15–1

When, during the course of operative therapy for cholelithiasis, exploration of the common bile duct is indicated, endoscopic examination of the common bile duct and its intrahepatic branches is a valuable adjunct to standard exploratory techniques. Instruments available for this purpose are of small caliber, may be rigid or flexible, and possess biopsy channels and accessories that permit diagnostic and therapeutic manipulation. This examination may be performed prior to other intraductal interventions or after standard ductal exploration. The instrument is introduced through the standard choledochotomy. Saline solution is continuously infused to keep the duct expanded. To adequately examine the distal portion of the bile duct, which curves to meet the duodenum, it is necessary to perform a Kocher maneuver and mobilize the second portion of the duodenum. Downward traction is applied to the second portion of the duodenum in order to straighten the duct and allow visualization of its most distal portion. In some cases the instrument may be passed through the ampulla into the duodenum. A stone identified in the distal duct may be captured in a basket and retrieved. The scope is slowly withdrawn while the lumen of the duct is inspected.

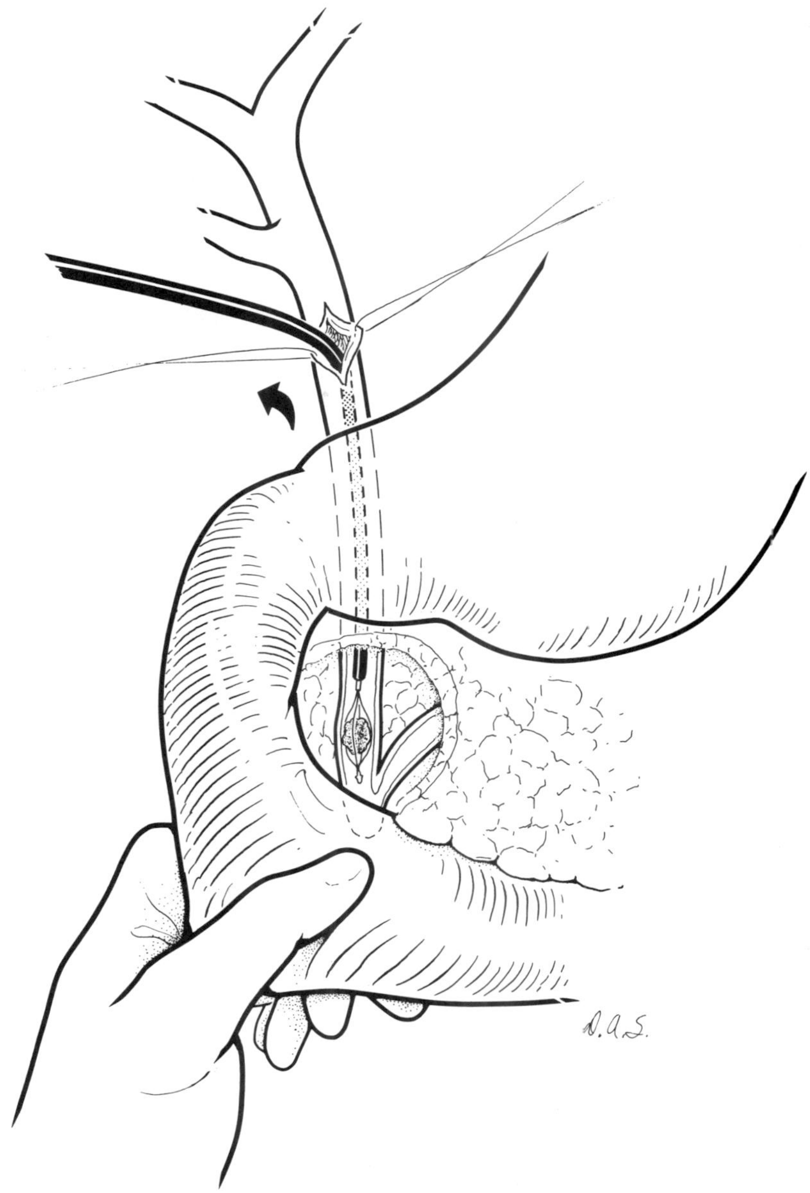
D.A.S.

PLATE 15–2

The choledochoscope is advanced into the proximal ductal system to the bifurcation of the ducts. The instrument is passed up each hepatic duct and side branches are inspected. When a stone is seen, a balloon catheter may be passed through the scope and maneuvered proximal to the stone **(A).**

With the balloon slightly inflated, the instrument is slowly withdrawn and the stone retrieved at the choledochotomy. Impacted or large stones may be treated with electrohydraulic or laser lithotripsy fibers passed through the channel of the choledochoscope **(B).**

A

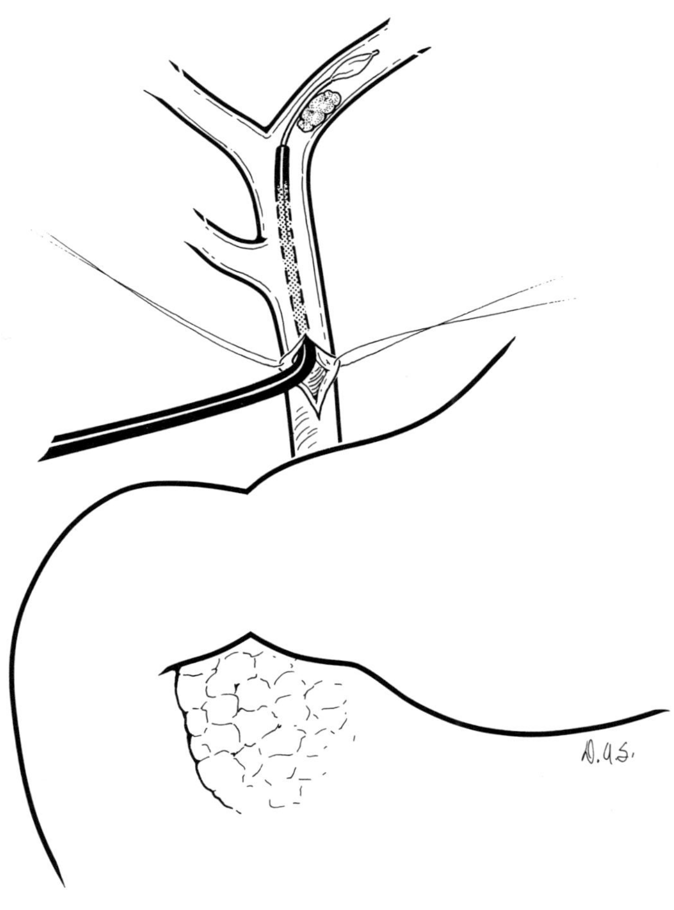

B

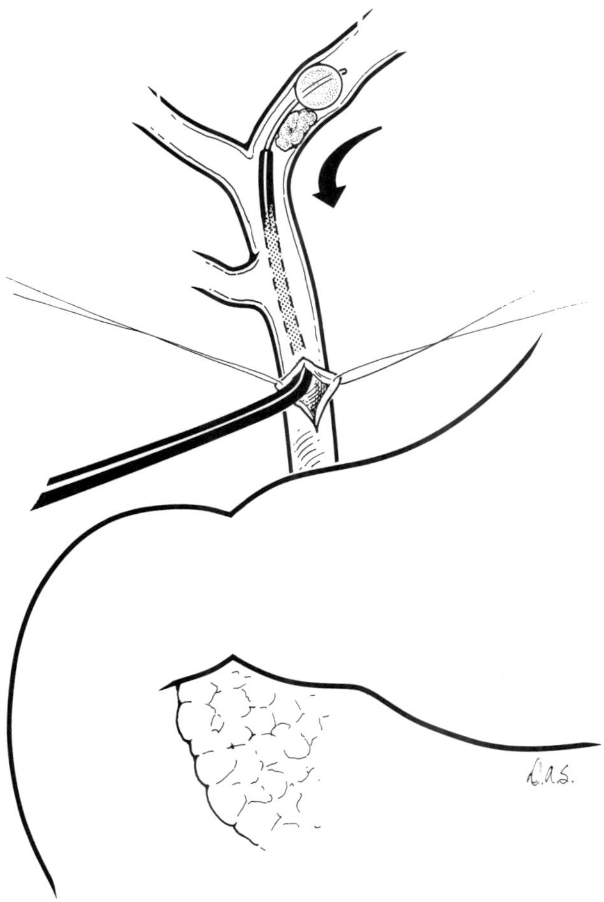

16

Laparoscopy

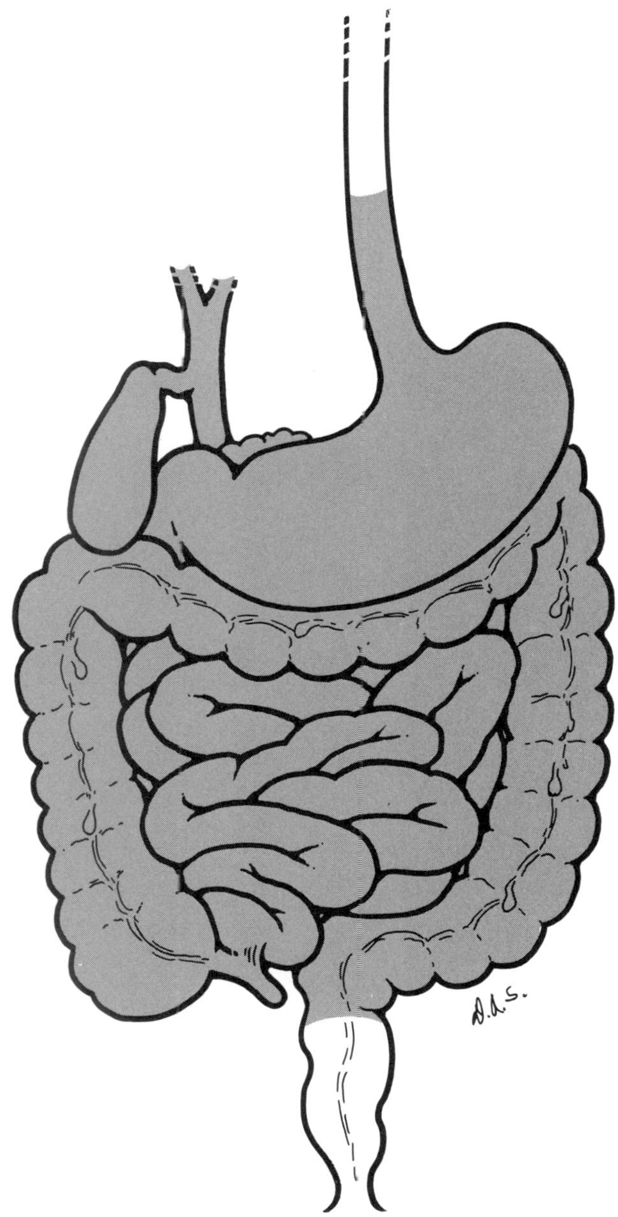

PLATE 16–1

The use of a telescope to examine the abdominal cavity is not new, having been introduced in the early part of this century. The safety and diagnostic accuracy of the method, referred to as laparoscopy or peritoneoscopy, has been well documented. The procedure has gained popularity among gynecologists, who have used the method with great success in the diagnosis and treatment of pelvic pathology. Gastroenterologists have used laparoscopy to evaluate the abdominal parietes, examine the liver, and to determine the etiology of ascites. Biopsy of small lesions may be performed under direct vision with great accuracy.

Laparoscopy may be performed utilizing local or general anesthesia. While diagnostic procedures are easily carried out with only mild sedation and local anesthetic, most therapeutic interventions require general anesthesia to assure patient comfort and safety. Prior to beginning the procedure, a nasogastric tube is usually inserted to empty the stomach and a urinary catheter to empty the bladder. These precautions help prevent inadvertent injury to abdominal viscera when instruments are introduced.

The patient is placed on the operating table in the supine position and the abdomen is prepared and draped in a sterile manner. The first step in performing laparoscopy is the establishment of satisfactory pneumoperitoneum, a cushion of gas that will permit safe entry of sharp instruments into the peritoneal cavity and enable the endoscopist to observe the viscera clearly. The table is tilted into the Trendelenburg position so that the patient's head is approximately 20 degrees down. This helps move most of the bowel cephalad, avoiding injury at the time of puncture. In most cases, a small skin incision is made at the inferior umbilical crease and a needle with a blunt, spring-loaded central stylet is slowly introduced through the abdominal wall and into the peritoneal cavity **(A).** Resistance to pressure will be felt to disappear and the central stylet will move inward when successful entry has been accomplished. Safe entry can also be assured by aspirating through the needle after insertion, making sure that no blood or intestinal content returns. A drop of saline solution instilled over the hub of the needle should fall quickly into the peritoneal cavity. Once the surgeon is satisfied that free entry has been accomplished, insufflation of gas may commence. Nitrous oxide and carbon dioxide have been successfully used to create pneumoperitoneum. While nitrous oxide may provide greater comfort for procedures performed under local anesthesia, it displays a greater potential to support combustion than does carbon dioxide. Thus, for most therapeutic procedures, carbon dioxide has been the gas of choice. Insufflation is begun slowly, at about 1 L/min.

After satisfactory pneumoperitoneum has been achieved, the insufflation needle is removed and the incision enlarged slightly. The subcutaneous tissue may be spread with a hemostat. A trocar with a sharp central stylet is then placed into the incision and rotated with a twisting motion while pressure is applied to insert it into the abdominal cavity **(B).** As soon as resistance disappears, pressure is stopped and the stylet removed. The tubing providing carbon dioxide for continued pneumoperitoneum is attached to the appropriate port on the trocar sleeve.

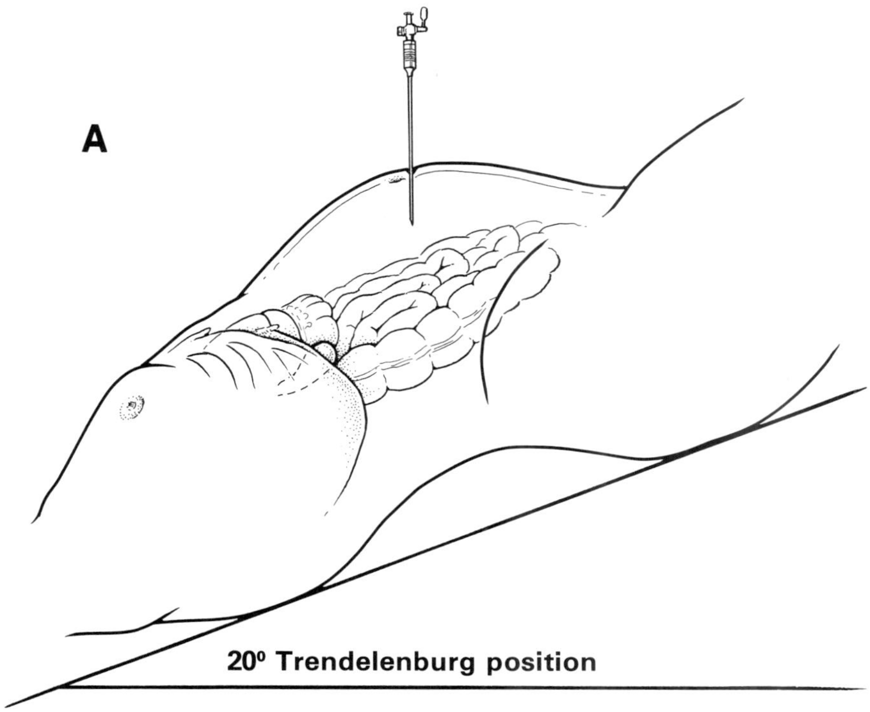
A
20° Trendelenburg position

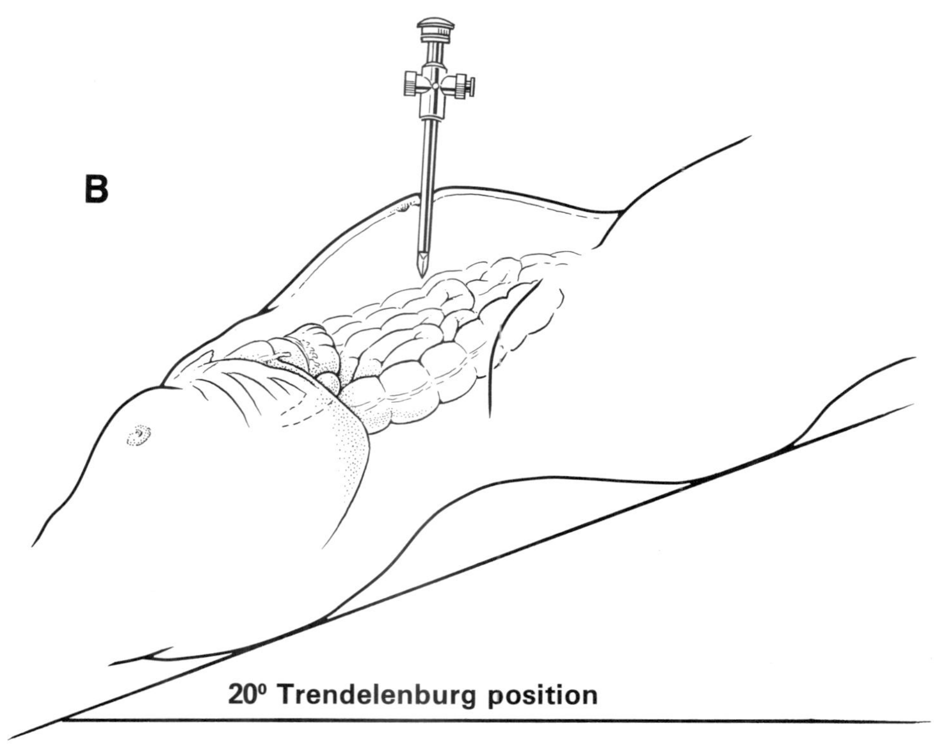
B
20° Trendelenburg position

PLATE 16–2

The laparoscope is introduced through the valve in the trocar sleeve. The light cable is attached to the instrument. Illustrated here is a video camera attached to the eyepiece of the laparoscope. The introduction of video technology has allowed all the members of the operating team to view the procedure and assist in its performance. While this adaptation is not necessary for strictly diagnostic laparoscopy, it is of crucial importance for most therapeutic endeavors.

The pelvis may be examined with the patient in the Trendelenburg position. In order to properly view the upper abdomen, the patient is turned to the reverse Trendelenburg position, causing the bowel to fall away from the stomach and undersurface of the liver. Additional trocars may be introduced under direct vision in order to manipulate organs and perform tissue sampling.

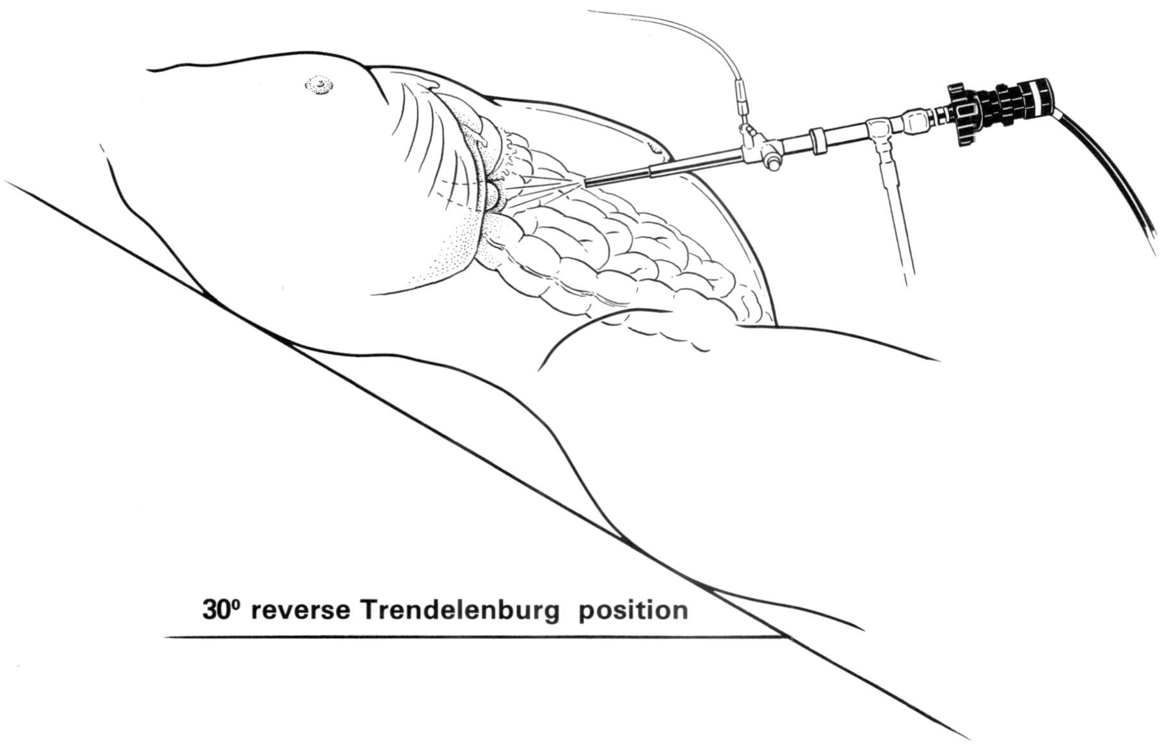
30° reverse Trendelenburg position

17

Laparoscopic Cholecystectomy

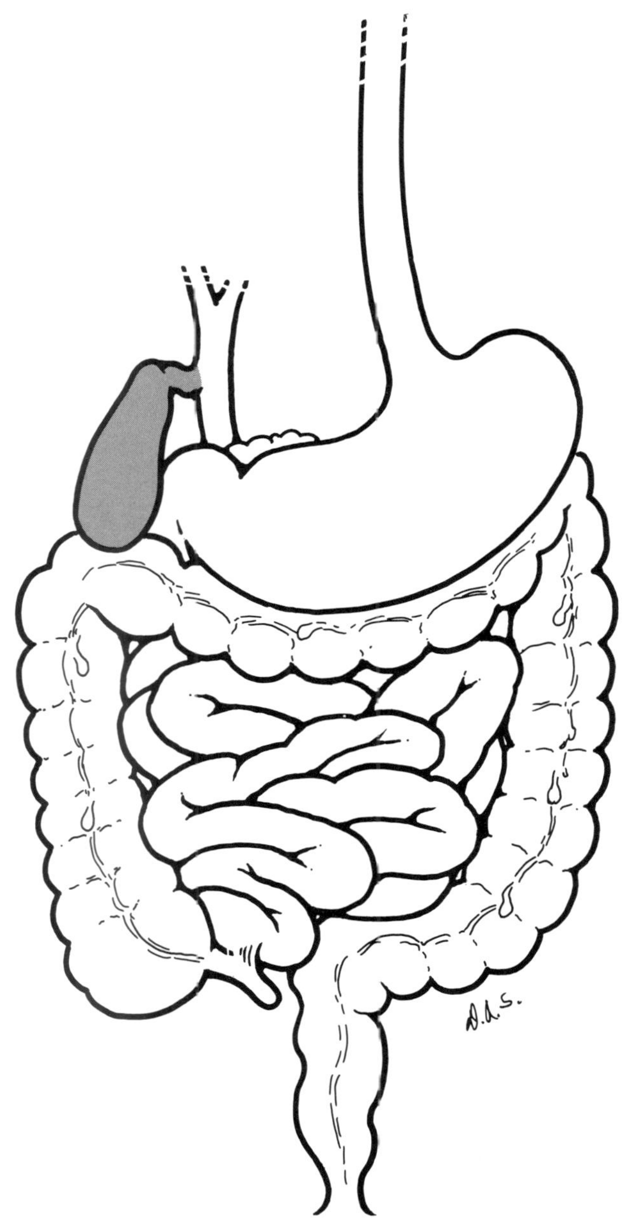

PLATE 17–1

Laparoscopic cholecystectomy was the first major therapeutic general surgical procedure performed with the laparoscope. Symptomatic cholecystolithiasis is the most common indication. The patient is prepared for the procedure just as for diagnostic laparoscopy and general anesthesia is used. Carbon dioxide is employed for establishment of the pneumoperitoneum. Video imaging is mandatory for a satisfactory team approach to the procedure. Generally, two video screens, one at each side of the patient, are employed so that the operators may look across the table to view the procedure.

As with standard diagnostic laparoscopy, the pneumoperitoneum needle and subsequent trocar are introduced at the umbilical crease. If concern exists as to safe entry of the pneumoperitoneum needle, the surgeon may choose to enter the abdomen by means of a small cutdown in this area. The trocar sheath may then be inserted into the peritoneal cavity under direct vision. For laparoscopic cholecystectomy, additional trocars are generally inserted in the epigastric region at the midline, in the midclavicular line near the costal margin, and in the anterior axillary line near the level of the umbilicus. The exact position of these punctures will vary based upon the surgeon's assessment after viewing the abdominal contents. This assessment is performed after insertion of the first trocar and prior to introduction of the others. Additional trocars may be inserted for retraction or manipulation as needed during the procedure.

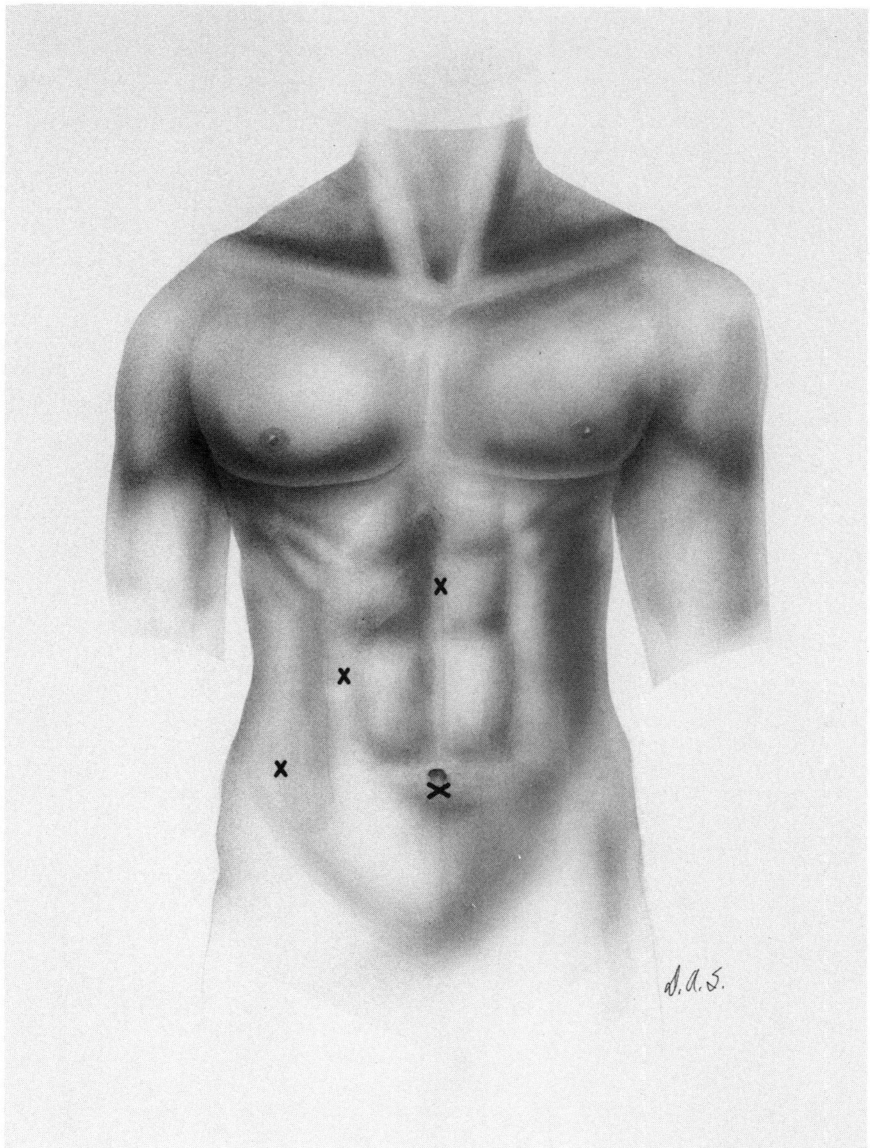

PLATE 17–2

After insertion of the desired trocars, a blunt forceps is introduced through the epigastric position and used to elevate the right lobe of the liver so that the gallbladder may be visualized. This forceps may then be used to grasp a portion of the gallbladder fundus and elevate it until it is properly grasped for retraction by a forceps from another port.

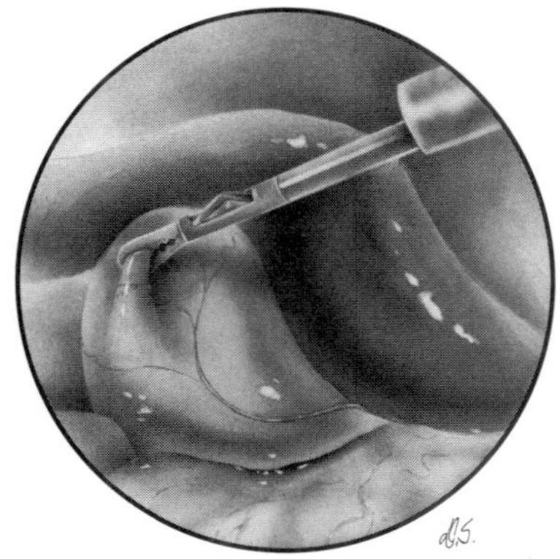

PLATE 17–3

A forceps with a ratcheted lock is introduced via the anterior axillary position and used to grasp the fundus of the gallbladder. Once the gallbladder is grasped, the forceps is advanced in a cephalad direction in order to retract the gallbladder and liver upward, exposing the portal structures **(A).**

Another grasping forceps is introduced through the port at the midclavicular line. This forceps is used to grasp the infundibulum of the gallbladder and distract it laterally and upward. This maneuver further exposes the portal structures and serves to straighten the cystic duct in preparation for its dissection **(B).**

A

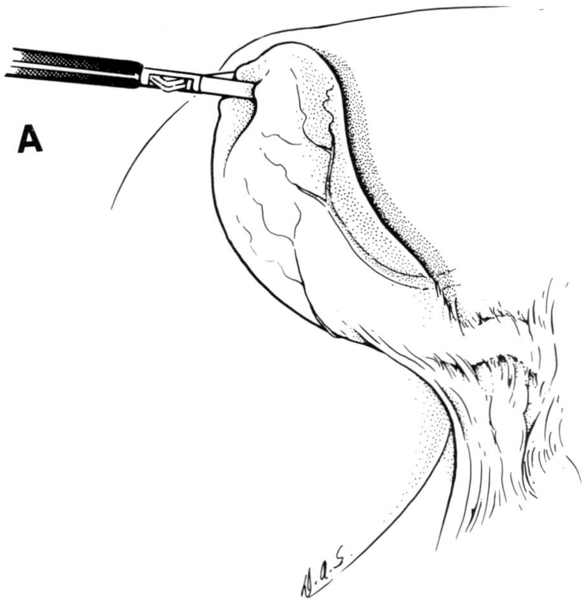

B

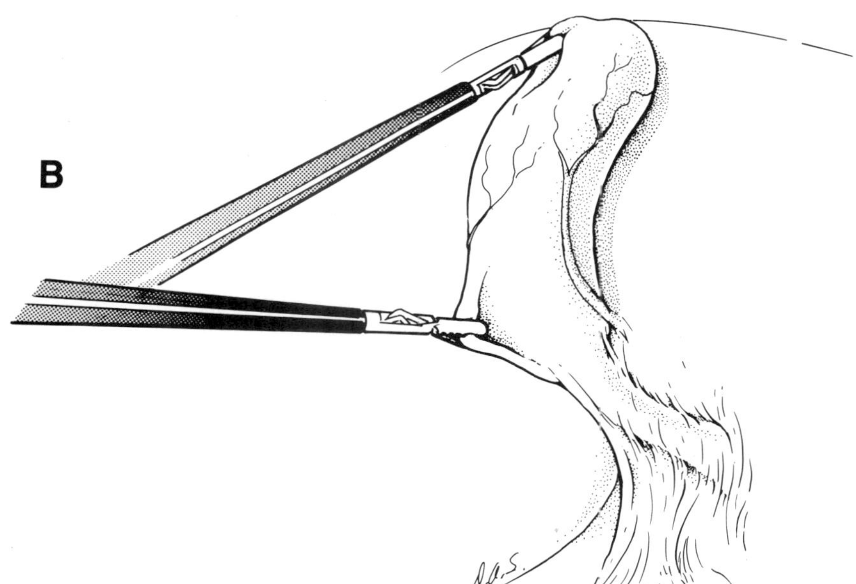

PLATE 17–4

The area of the cystic duct and artery is covered by the tissue of the gastrohepatic ligament. Also, adhesions may exist between the duodenum and gallbladder. This tissue is gently grasped with a smooth forceps passed through the epigastric portal and teased downward and away from the gallbladder, bringing the cystic duct into view **(A).**

The cystic duct is dissected free by blunt dissection. It is best to perform this dissection as close to the gallbladder as possible to avoid injury to the common bile duct. A variety of straight and curved forceps are available for this dissection, as well as dissection hooks that can be used to surround the duct and strip connective tissue away from it **(B).**

Once isolated, clips may be applied to the cystic duct. It is usually preferable to perform cystic duct cholangiography prior to division of the duct; this helps to assure that there are no overlooked common bile duct calculi and that any unsuspected anatomic variations are identified. In preparation for the cholangiogram a clip is applied across the cystic duct, close to its junction with the gallbladder **(C).**

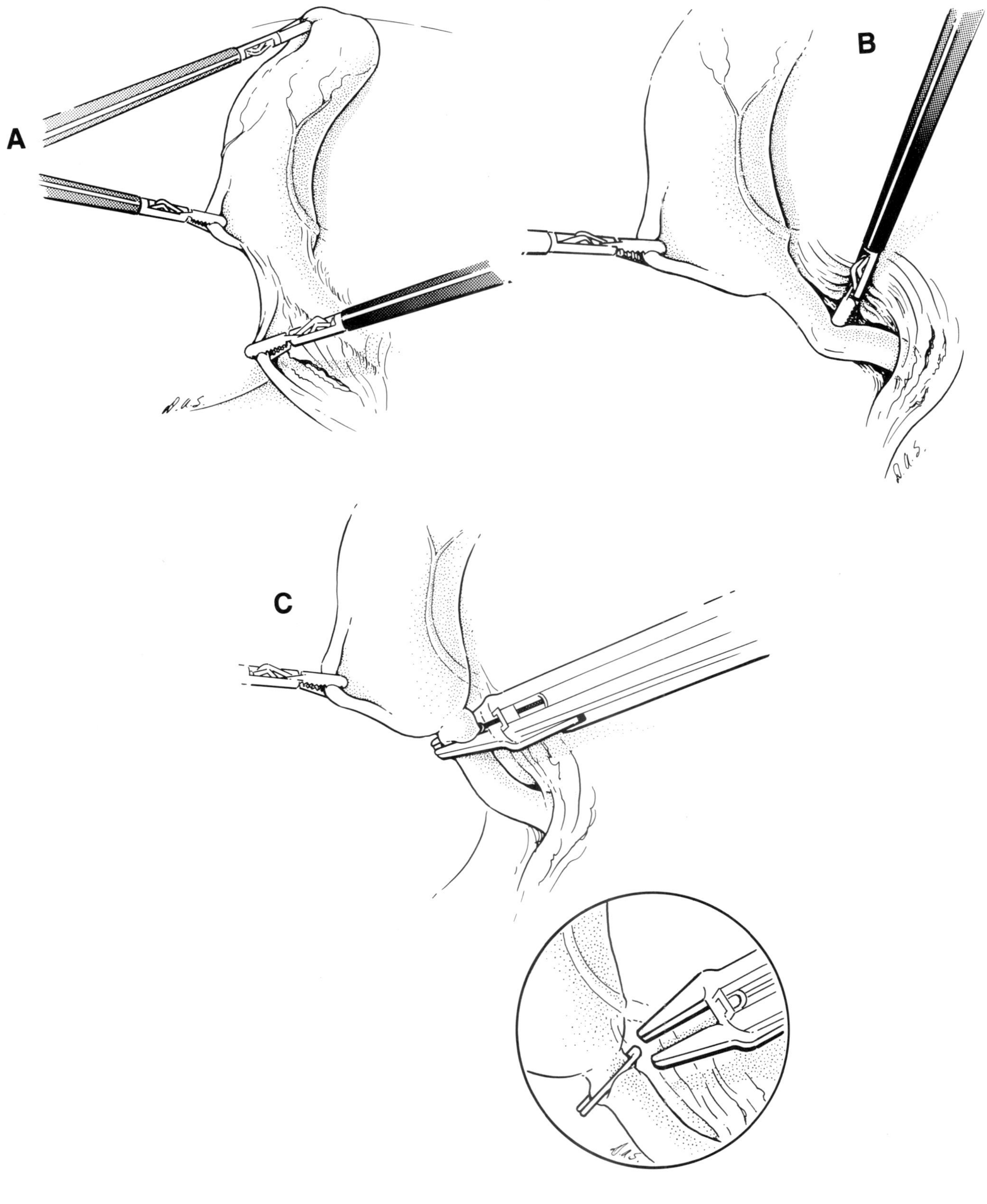
A
B
C

PLATE 17–5

A variety of methods may be employed for insertion of a cannula into the cystic duct. Demonstrated here is the passage of the cannula through a clamp designed to grasp the duct and prevent reflux during injection of contrast material.

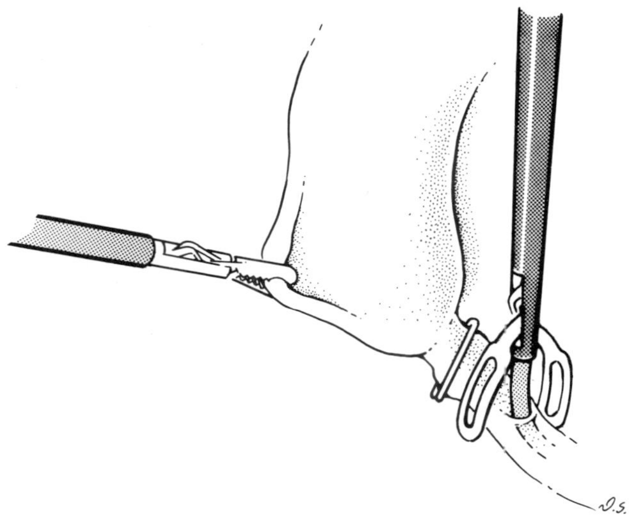

PLATE 17–6

After completion of a cholangiogram, two clips are applied to the proximal portion of the cystic duct and it is divided. In like fashion, the cystic artery is exposed by blunt dissection and followed to its junction with the gallbladder. Two clips are applied to its proximal portion and one distally prior to division of the artery.

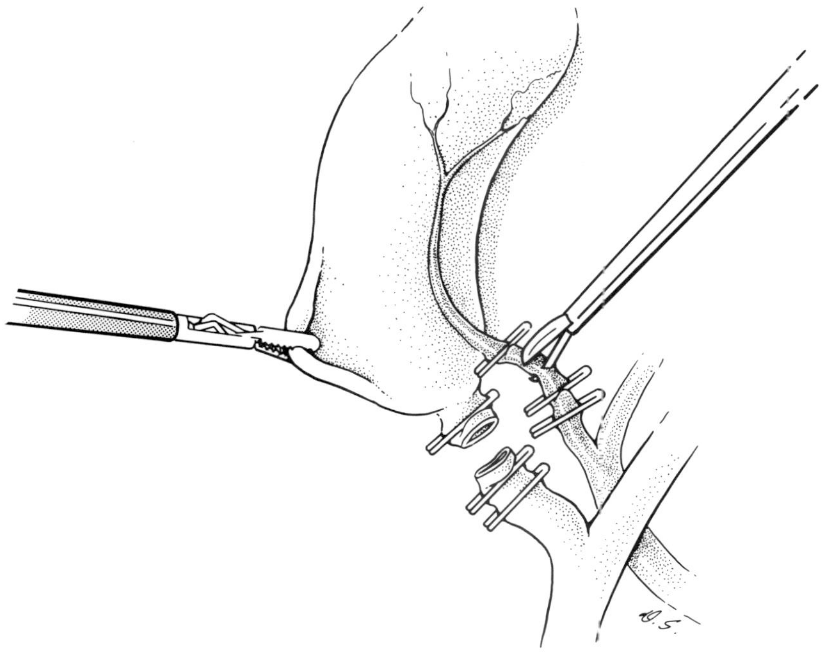

PLATE 17–7

Traction is applied to the infundibulum of the gallbladder and efforts proceed to remove it from its bed. The laser or cautery may be used to divide the attachments of the gallbladder to the liver. Demonstrated here is the use of a hook dissector and cautery. Pure coagulation current is used and most effective sectioning of tissue occurs when tension is provided by lateral retraction of the gallbladder. The tissue planes are generally evident and dissection is performed from the infundibular area toward the fundus, working alternately on one side of the gallbladder and then the other.

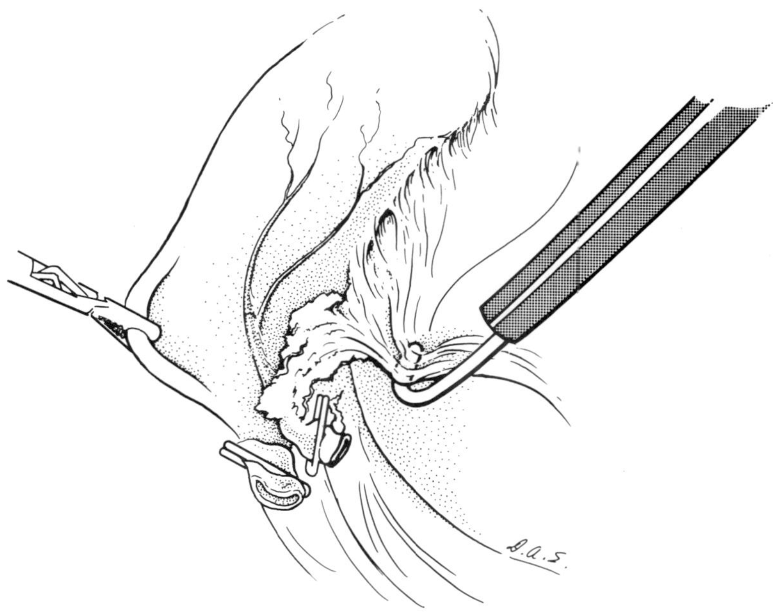
D.A.S.

PLATE 17–8

When only a small tongue of tissue remains to be divided, the surgeon should use the gallbladder as a retractor to lift the liver and examine the raw surfaces of the gallbladder bed for bleeding or bile leakage. If such areas are identified they should be dealt with at this time by the application of cautery, endoscopic ligatures, or clips. The bed should be irrigated and then suctioned free of fluid. Finally, the remaining attachments of the gallbladder to the liver may be divided **(A).**

Once free, the gallbladder is held over the liver. The patient is turned once again to the Trendelenburg position and the pool of fluid over the liver removed by suction. This may help to reduce postoperative discomfort. The laparoscope and camera are then transferred from the umbilical to the epigastric position. A large grasping forceps is introduced through the umbilical port and used to grasp the gallbladder near its cystic duct stump. This is its smallest portion and most ideal for extraction **(B).** Under direct observation via the laparoscope, the gallbladder is withdrawn from the abdomen and slightly into the umbilical trocar with a twisting motion. No attempt is made to remove it completely through the trocar; rather, once a portion of the gallbladder neck has entered the shaft of the trocar, the trocar sleeve is itself removed from the abdomen **(C).** The gallbladder is grasped with a clamp when it appears at skin level and slowly teased from the abdomen. If removal is difficult, the neck of the gallbladder may be opened and the contents suctioned. If difficulty still exists, the fascial incision may be enlarged just enough to permit passage of the gallbladder. Following removal of the gallbladder, the pneumoperitoneum is evacuated and the incisions irrigated before closure.

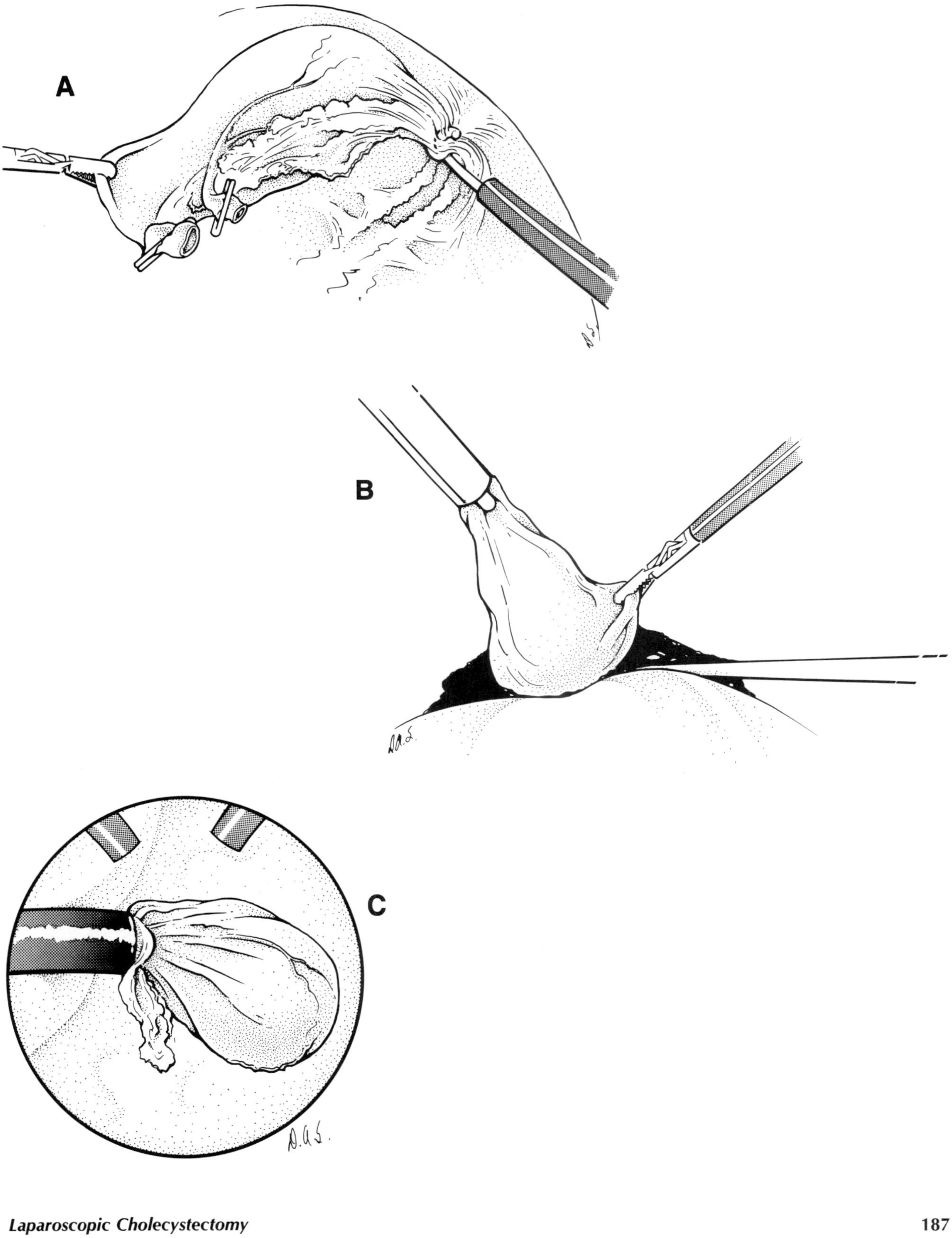
A
B
C

18

Laparoscopic Appendectomy

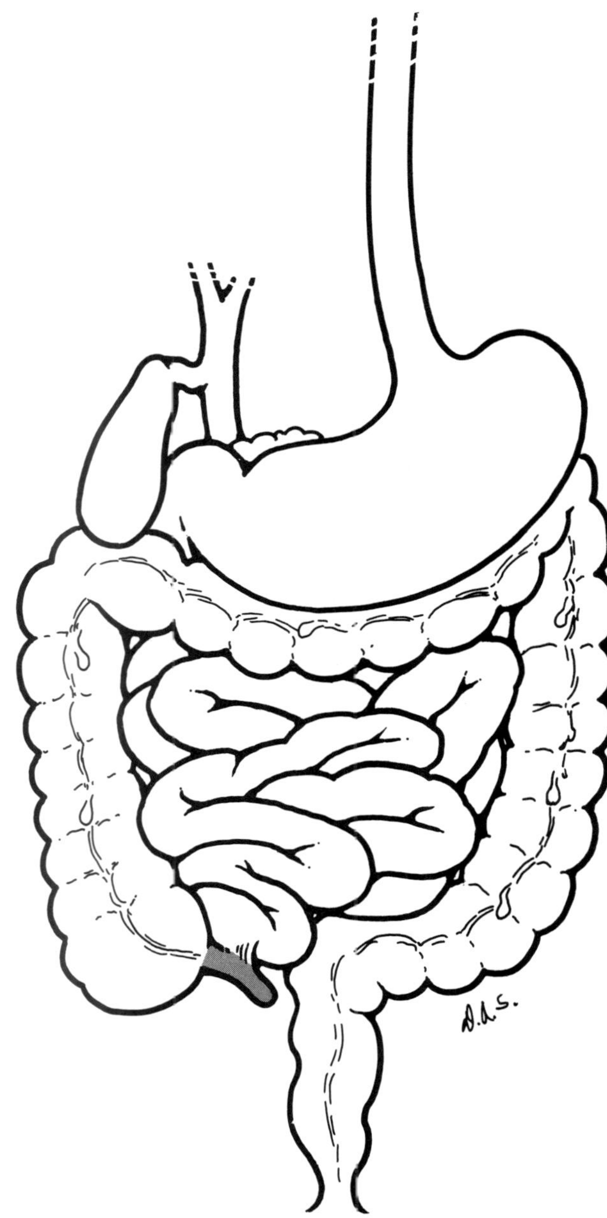

PLATE 18–1

Laparoscopic removal of the appendix is a feasible alternative to laparotomy in many cases. It may be particularly useful when, in the evaluation of equivocal cases by laparoscopy, the appendix is found to be inflamed. The initial stages in the laparoscopy are identical with those described for laparoscopic cholecystectomy. The initial pneumoperitoneum and trocar access are established through the umbilical crease. The patient is turned to the Trendelenburg position and additional trocars are placed. Common insertion sites include the suprapubic midline, the right iliac region, and the right anterior axillary line at the umbilical level. Blunt forceps are used to manipulate the bowel until the right colon, cecum, and appendix are visualized. In this illustration, a smooth forceps is used to grasp and elevate the appendix, exposing its mesoappendix **(A).** Sometimes an additional forceps can be used to grasp the cecum and retract it cephalad.

Dissecting forceps are used to dissect pedicles of the mesoappendix in preparation for their ligation and division **(B).** Traction upon the appendix facilitates this dissection.

Sequentially, the pedicles of the mesoappendix are isolated, clipped twice proximally and once distally, and divided. When the base of the appendix is reached, loose areolar tissue is teased away from the area and a blunt forceps applied across the appendix at its base in preparation for the application of a ligature at this point. A pretied endoscopic ligature is passed over the tip of the appendix and positioned at its base **(C).** The ligature is then tied down and cut.

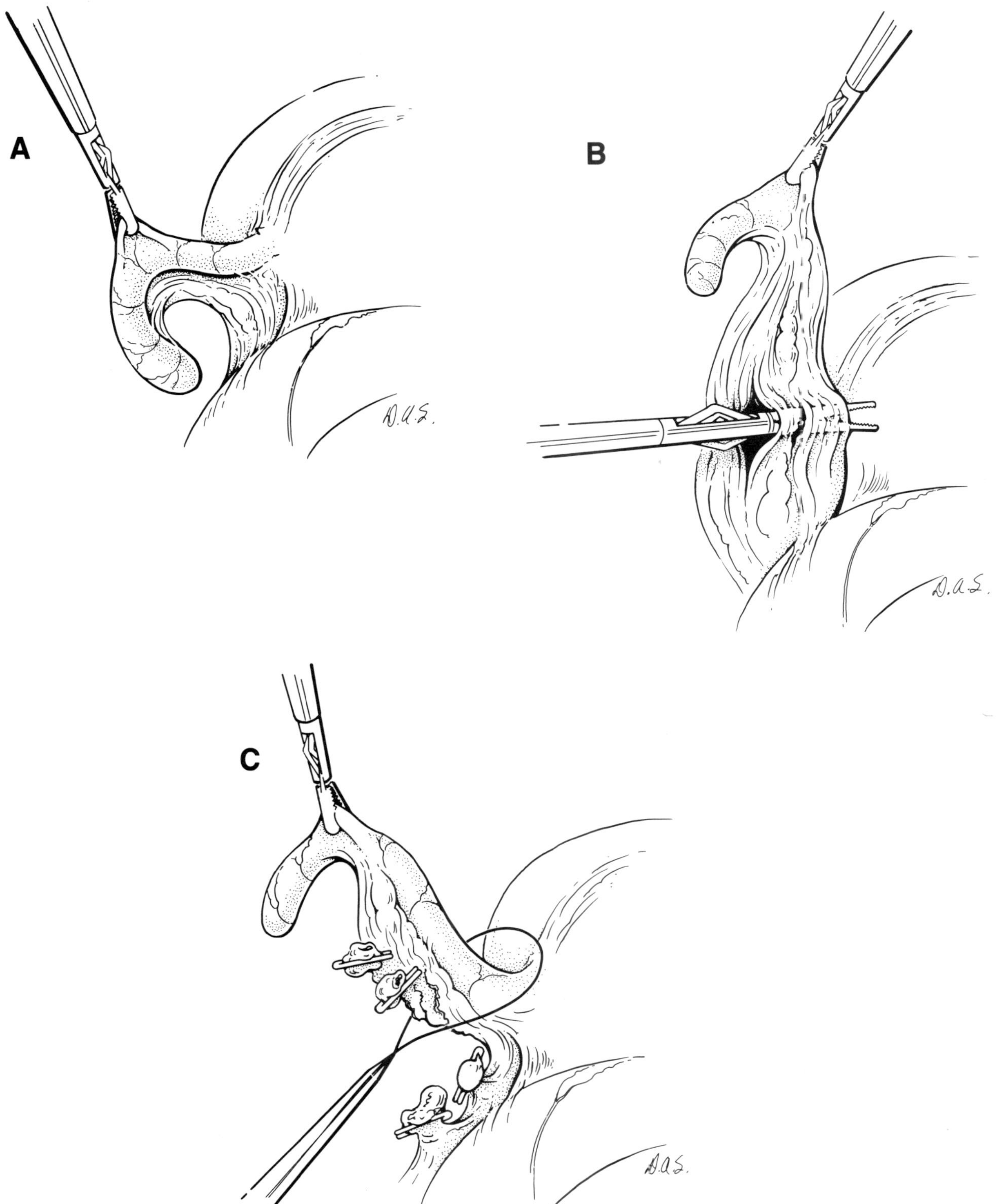
A
B
C

PLATE 18–2

Two additional ligatures are applied: one next to the first ligature at the appendiceal base and a final ligature more distally. The appendix is then transected between the two most distal ligatures **(A),** leaving two ties on the appendiceal stump.

With the excised appendix held in the visual field, the mucosa of the remaining stump is cauterized with the hook coagulator **(B).** The abdomen is irrigated and the fluid removed with suction. The appendix is then removed through one of the trocar sites. The incisions are irrigated and closed.

A

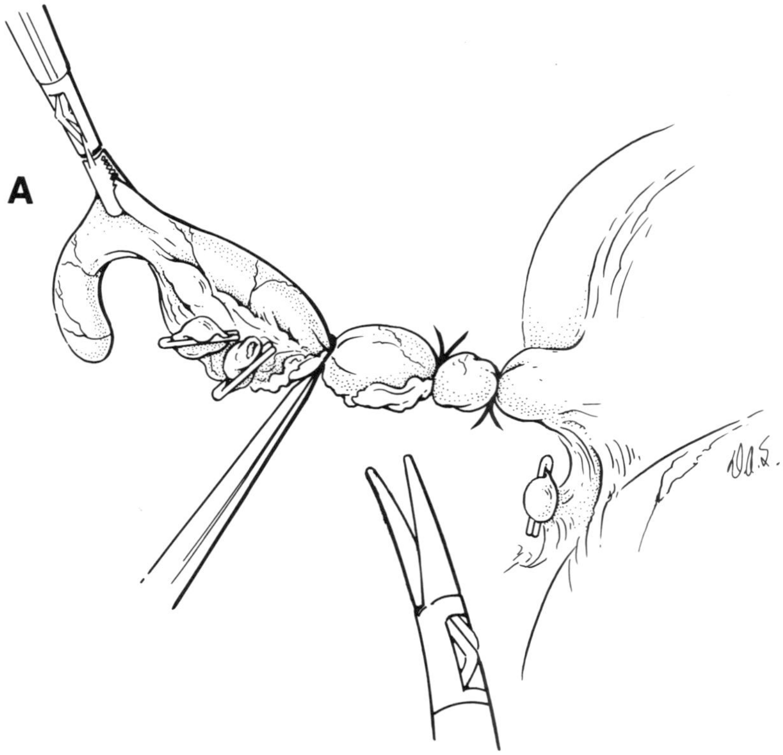

B

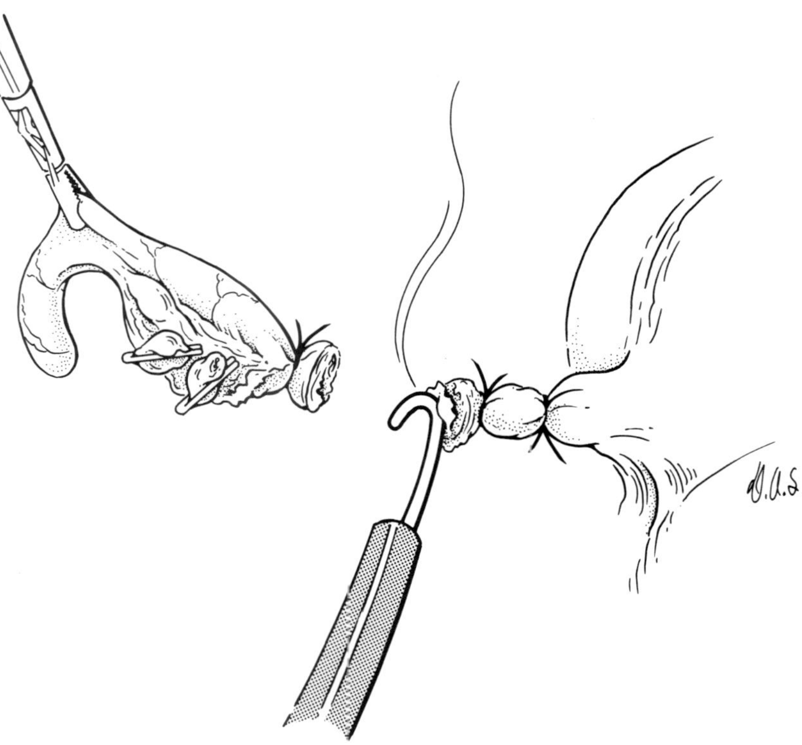

19

Colonoscopy

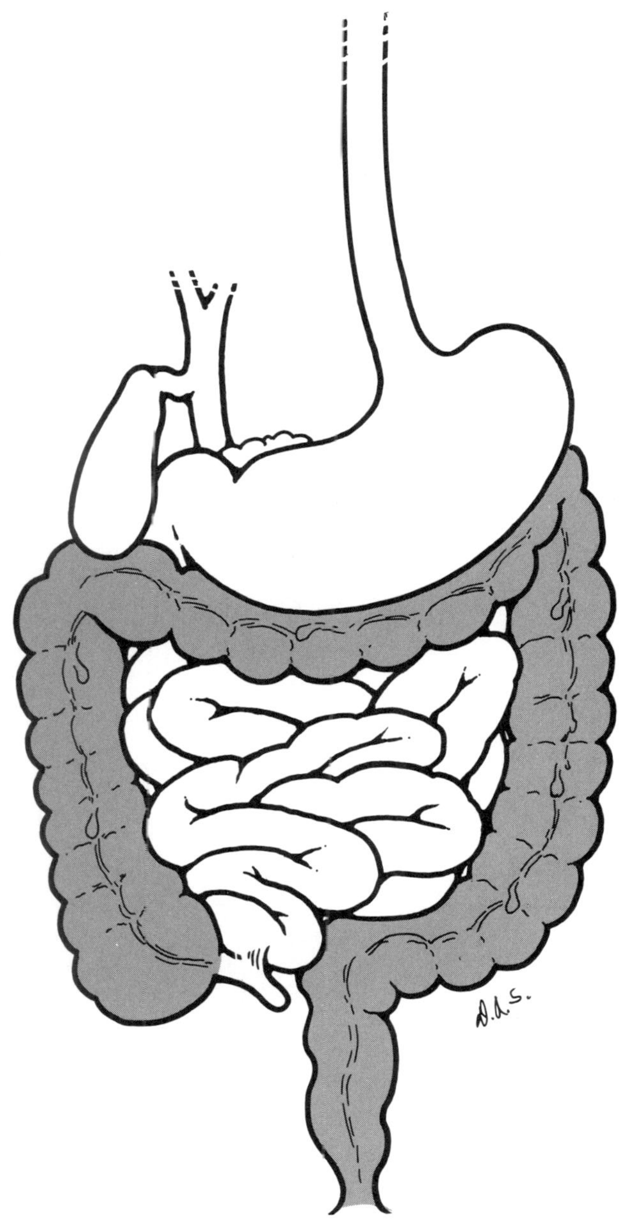

PLATE 19–1

Colonoscopy is perhaps the most frequently performed endoscopic procedure. It has revolutionized the diagnosis and treatment of colonic disease and improvements in instrumentation have made its performance far less formidable a task. Adequate mechanical preparation of the colon is imperative prior to the examination. Intravenous sedation is commonly used to enhance patient comfort.

The patient is placed in the left lateral decubitus position. A careful rectal examination is performed prior to insertion of the instrument. The endoscopist may choose to wear two gloves on the hand inserting the instrument, removing the outer one after introduction of the endoscope. The instrument is well lubricated and held about an inch from its tip. The tip is then placed on the patient's perineal body and pulled slowly backward while applying pressure toward the anus. This permits the side of the instrument's tip to dilate the anus gradually as it approaches and reduces trauma to the anal canal as the colonoscope is inserted.

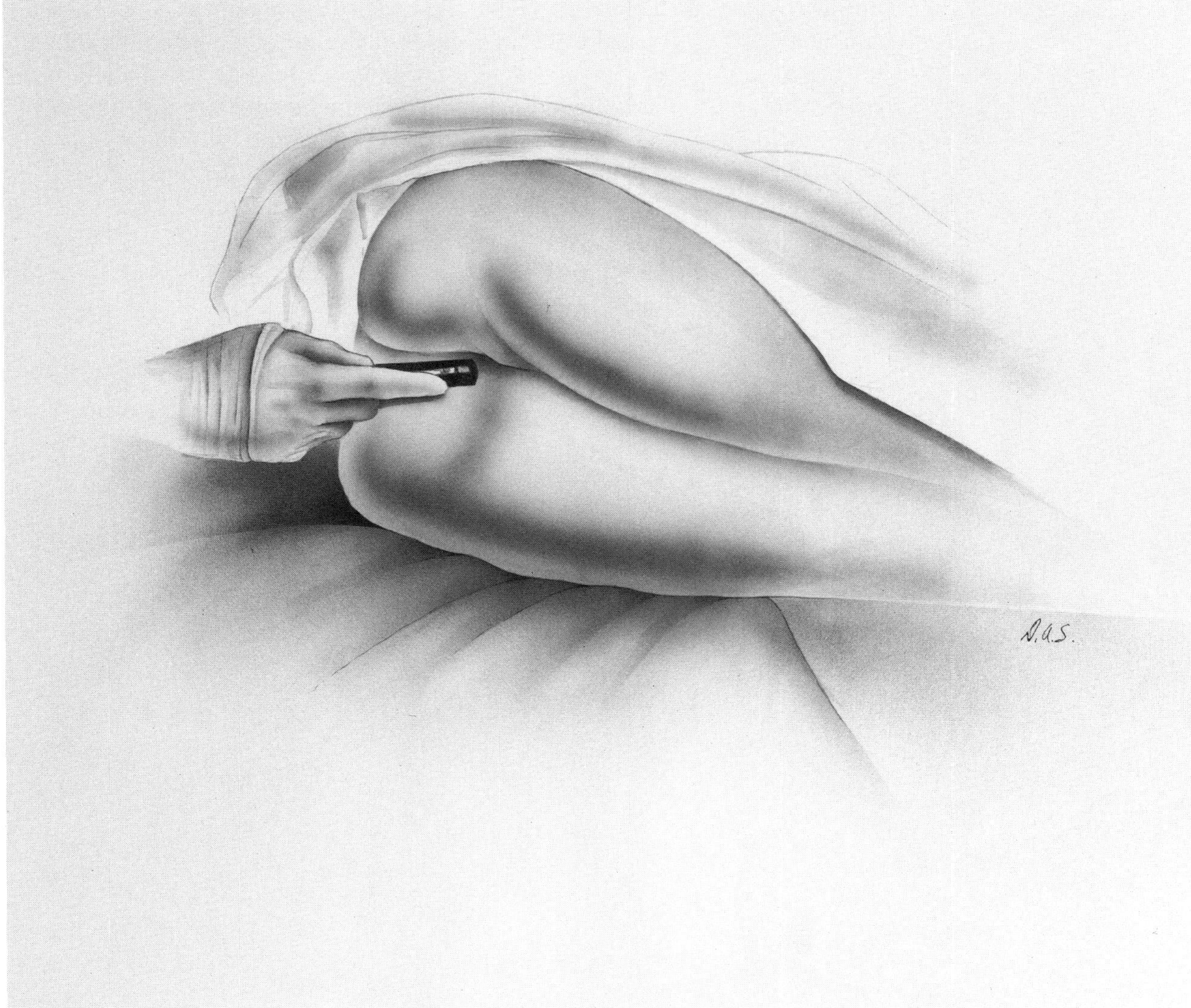

PLATE 19–2

After insertion of the colonoscope into the rectum, air is insufflated and any accumulated debris is washed from the lens. Insufflation should be continued only until the rectal lumen is expanded. Excessive or continuous insufflation of air produces patient discomfort and renders colonic intubation more difficult. In the rectum, the valves appear as semilunar folds, in an alternating fashion. The mucosa should be smooth with prominent vascular markings. Rectal vasculature is typically more prominent than that seen in the rest of the colon.

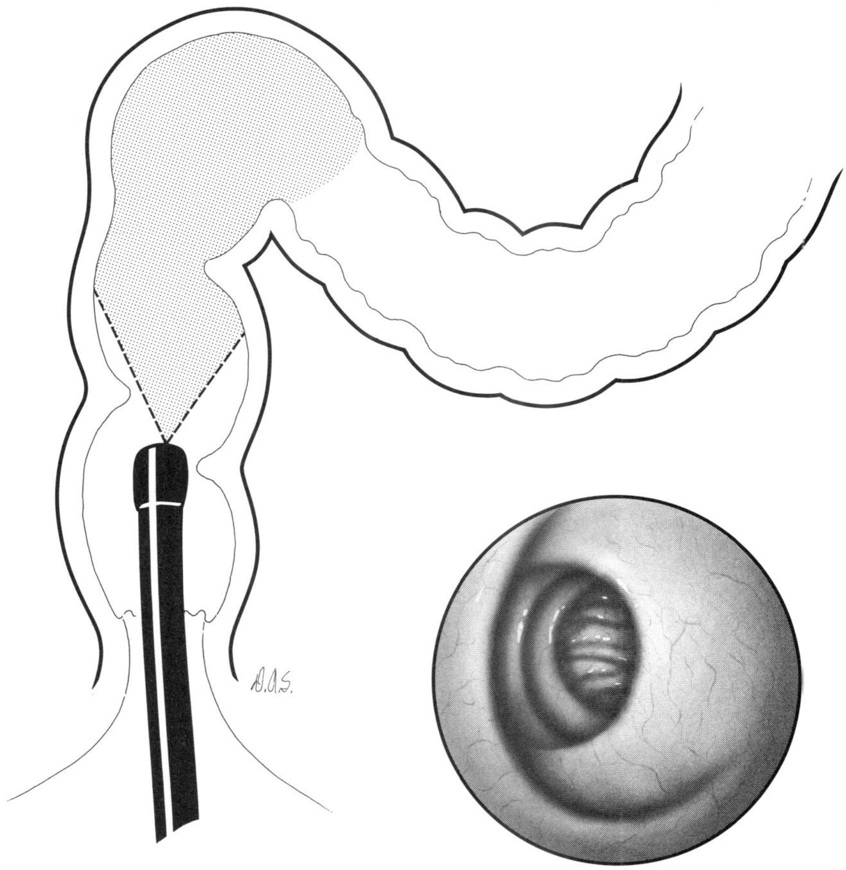

PLATE 19–3

The instrument is advanced slowly while the endoscopist continuously seeks the lumen. As the colon turns, the entire lumen may not be visible at one time and the endoscopist may use indirect signs to help localize the correct course. Highlights of reflected light appearing on the edges of the colonic folds help point the way. The concavity of the folds points toward the direction of the intestinal lumen. It is useful to twist the shaft of the instrument as it is advanced, as this may expose the lumen and help in advancing the instrument. When the lumen is not apparent, no attempt should be made to advance the instrument. Although early texts described the technique of pushing the scope inward along the mucosa as long as the mucosa moved by ("slide by"), this technique is apt to lead to perforation and should be avoided if possible. Advancement of the colonoscope with direct observation of the lumen is most preferable.

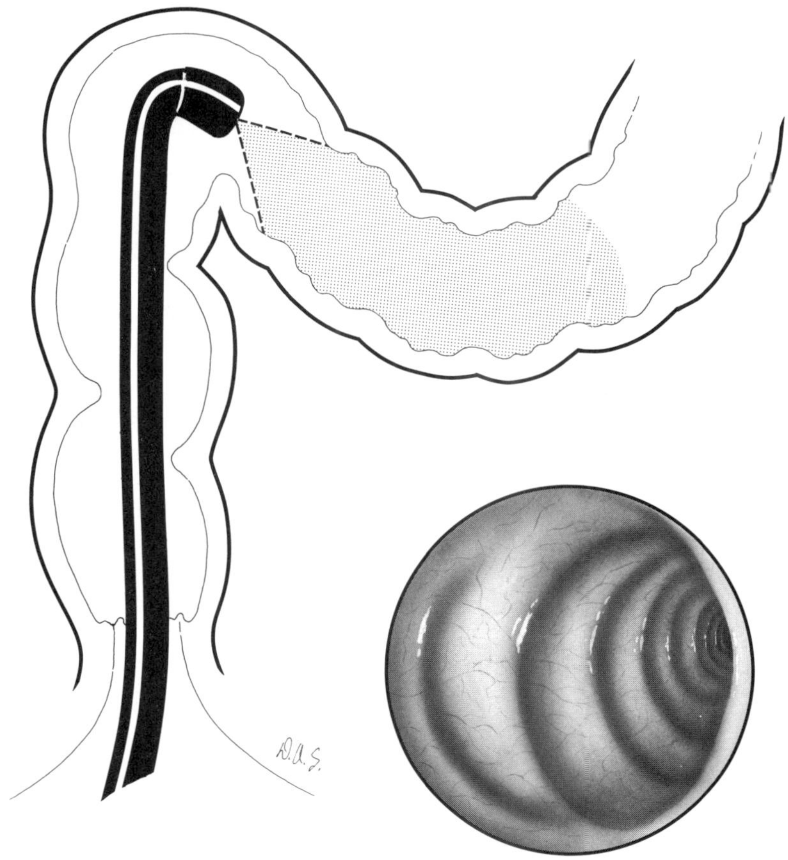

PLATE 19–4

The colonoscope is slowly advanced through the turns of the sigmoid colon, passing one fold at a time **(A).** Loops frequently form in the shaft of the instrument as it is inserted more deeply. The patient may experience discomfort, indicating that the mesentery of the bowel is being stretched. Excessive pressure may lead to perforation of the colon at the point where a bowing of the shaft occurs; thus, the endoscopist should remain cognizant of the patient's complaints and use them as a guide while applying pressure to the shaft of the endoscope.

When loop formation leads to excessive pain or the inability to advance the instrument, it is useful to pull back on the shaft of the scope and straighten it, removing the loops. This is sometimes facilitated by hooking the tip of the instrument around a turn and then withdrawing the shaft of the colonoscope **(B).** Attempts to advance the instrument may then be resumed.

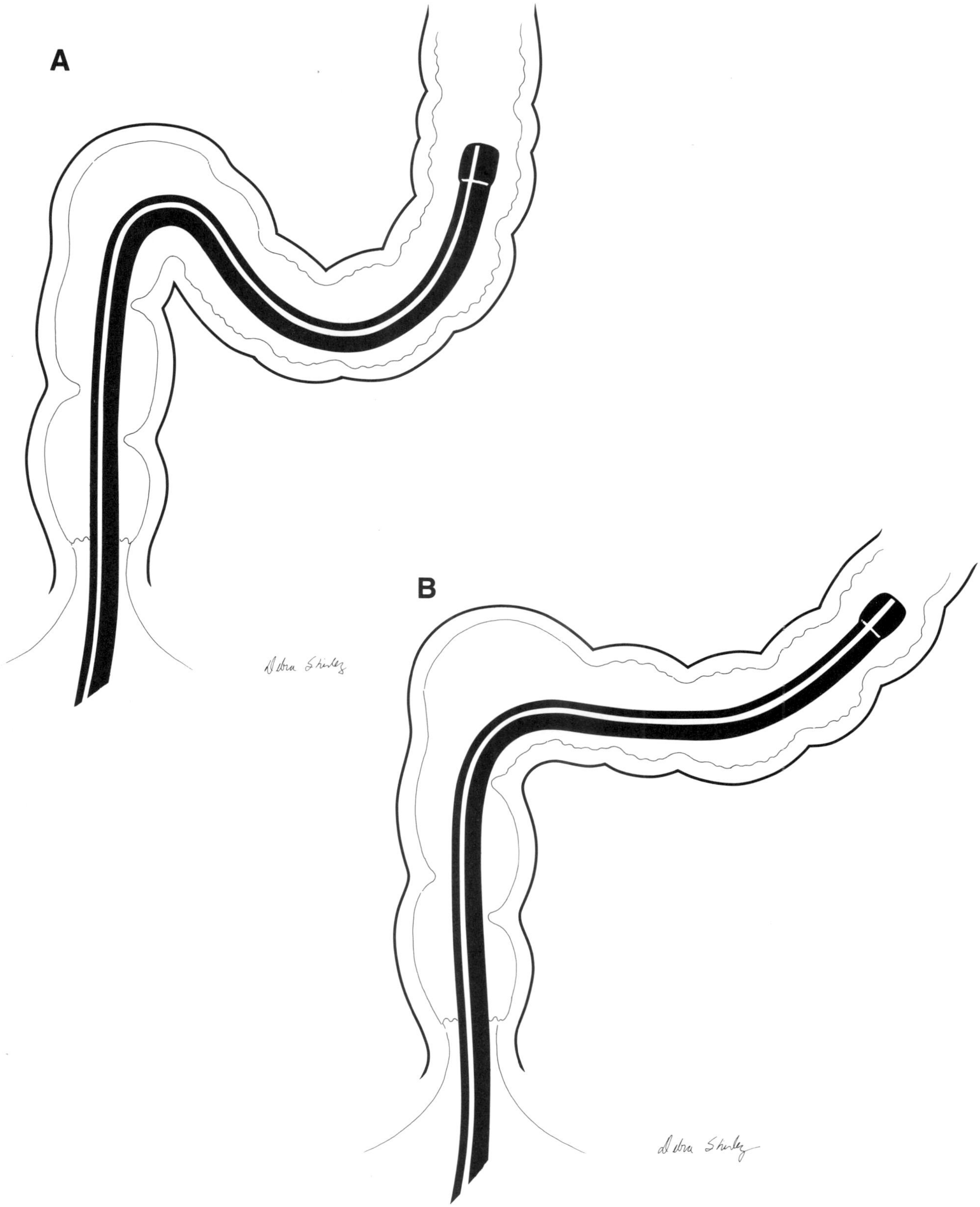
A
B

PLATE 19–5

The descending colon usually appears as a long, round tube with concentric, round folds. It is relatively straight and most of its lumen can be visualized in one view. This figure also demonstrates how straightening of the colonic loops acts to telescope the redundant colon onto the shaft of the instrument.

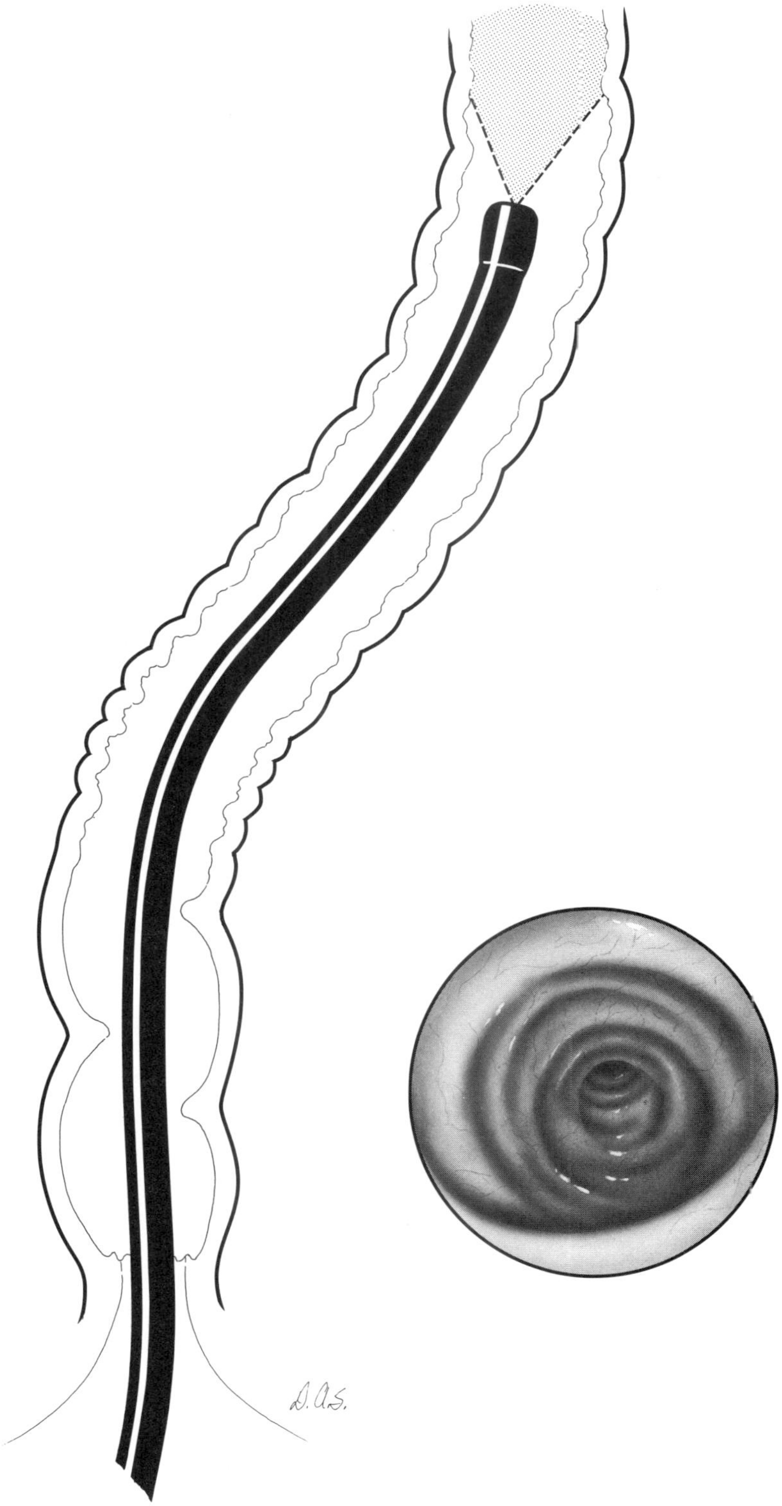
D.A.S.

PLATE 19–6

At the proximal end of the descending colon a turn to the left usually brings the lumen of the transverse colon into view. Once the tip of the instrument enters the transverse colon it is useful to again pull back on the shaft of the scope and straighten it prior to advancing further.

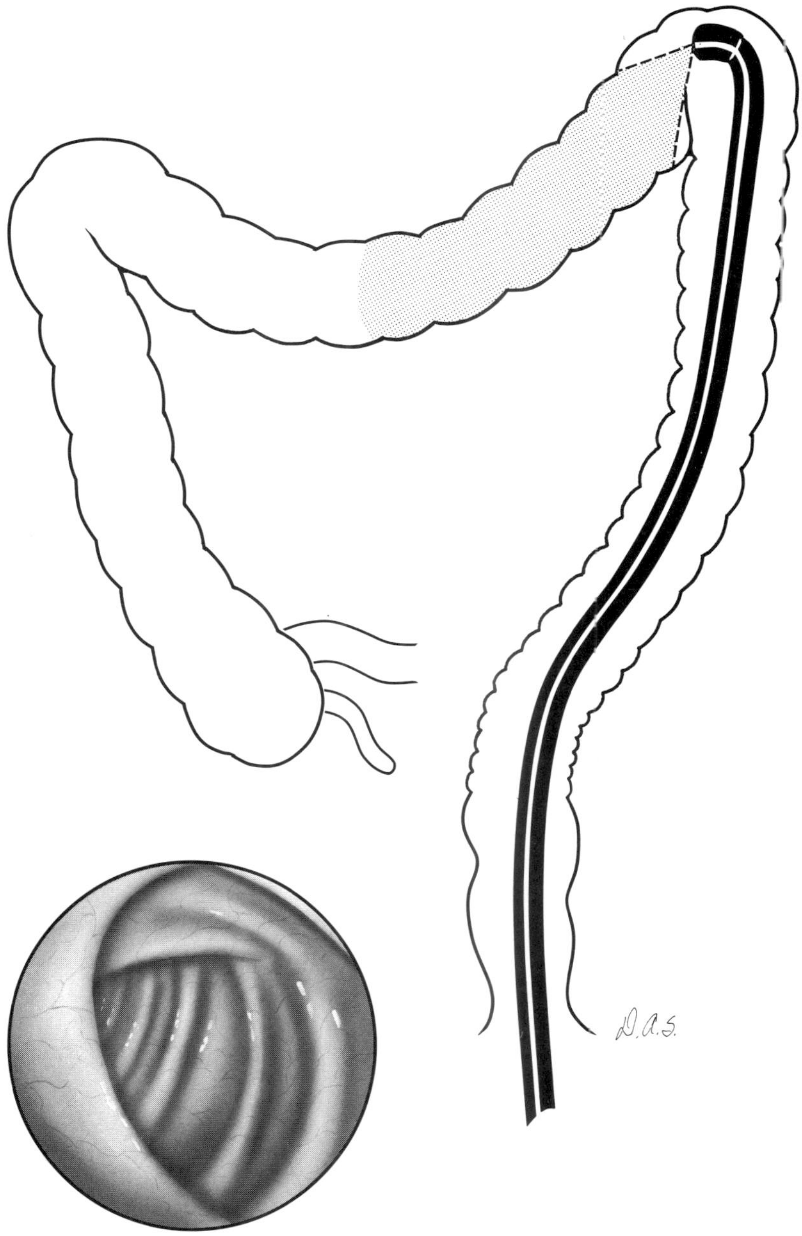
D.A.S.

PLATE 19–7

Triangular haustral folds clearly identify the transverse colon. This colonic segment is easily traversed by advancing the shaft of the colonoscope. Loops tend to form again as the instrument proceeds.

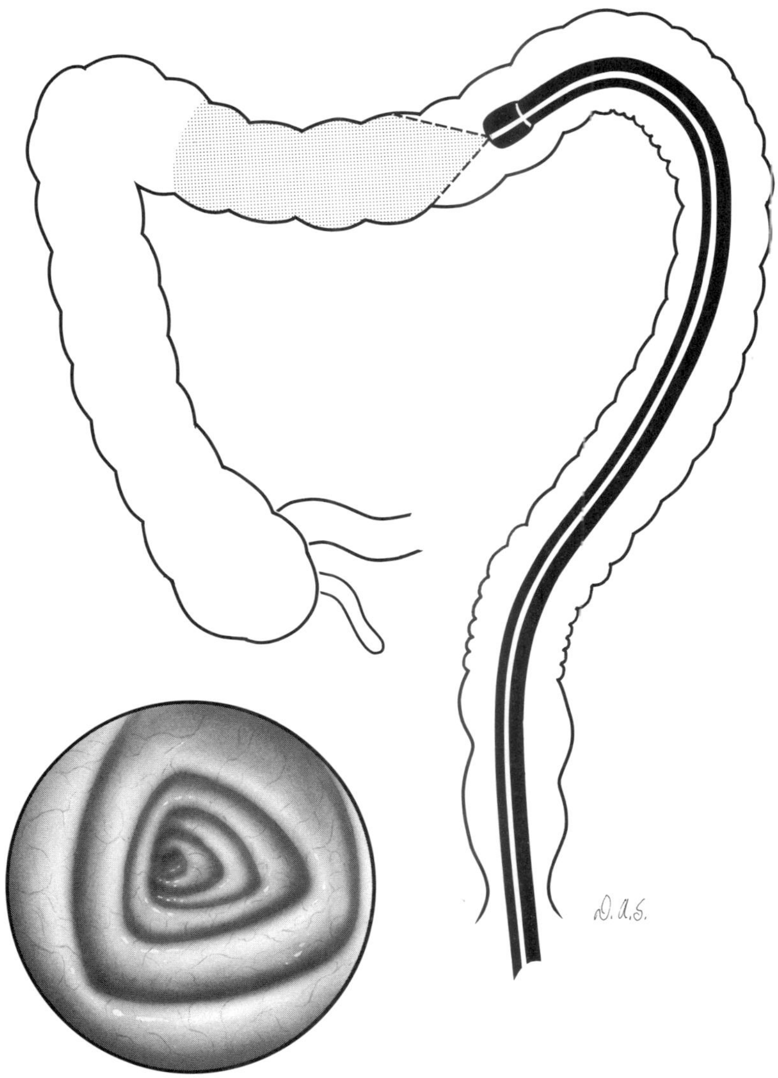
D.A.S.

PLATE 19–8

At the hepatic flexure the endoscopist will notice the bluish hue of the liver adjacent to the colonic wall. Generally, a turn to the left signals the entrance into the right colon. Frequently, it is difficult to advance the scope into the ascending colon by direct insertion of the shaft. One may encounter paradoxical motion: the tip of the instrument moves backward as the shaft is inserted. This phenomenon alerts the examiner that loops again exist and must be dealt with. Two maneuvers are possible. Most often effective is withdrawing the scope with a jiggling motion in an attempt to further telescope the colon onto its shaft and remove loops. An alternative, but more risky, approach is to continue to apply pressure to the loop, carefully monitoring the patient's response. If the instrument responds and the tip advances, this method, pushing through the loop, may be successful.

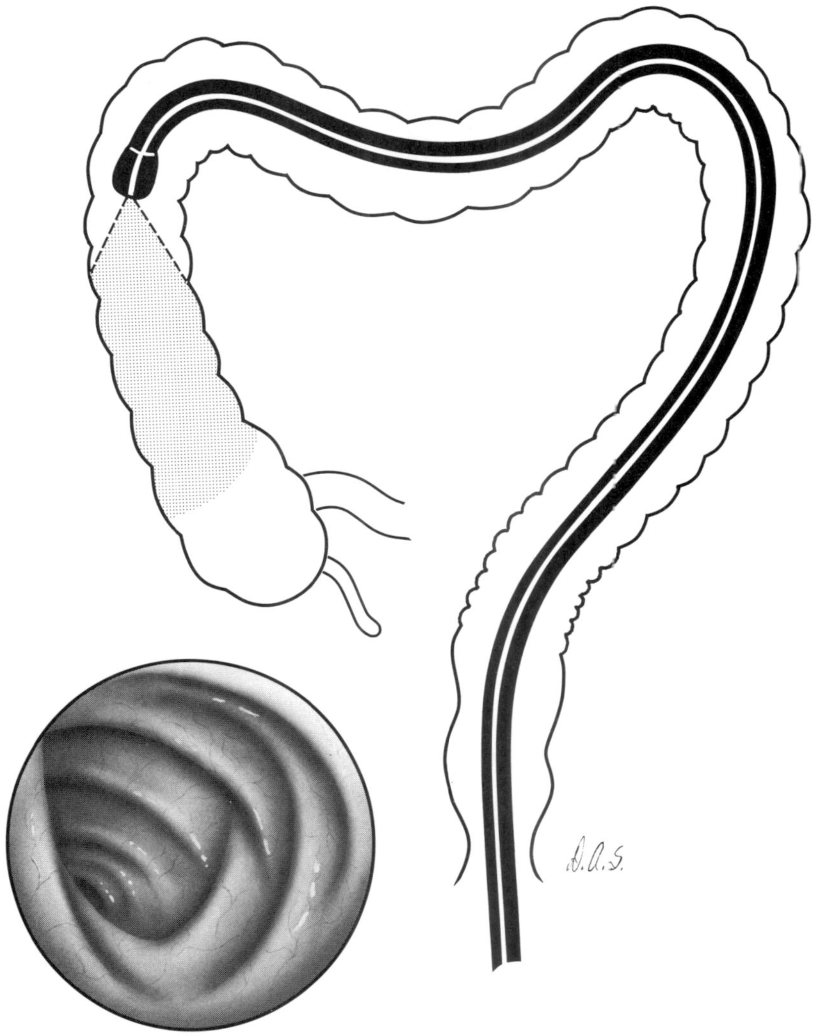

PLATE 19–9

When the cecum has been reached, it may be identified by its anatomic features. These include a convergence of the colonic tenia with the central appendiceal orifice, the thickened, liplike folds of the ileocecal valve, and transillumination of the abdominal wall in the right lower quadrant of the abdomen. Once again, withdrawal of the redundant loops will enhance patient comfort and often assist in reaching the most proximal portion of the cecum.

Although insertion of the instrument is the most challenging part of the procedure, perhaps the most important part of the examination is careful observation of the colonic walls upon removal of the scope. This should be done by slow withdrawal of the shaft, while the tip of the endoscope is rotated to observe all mucosal surfaces.

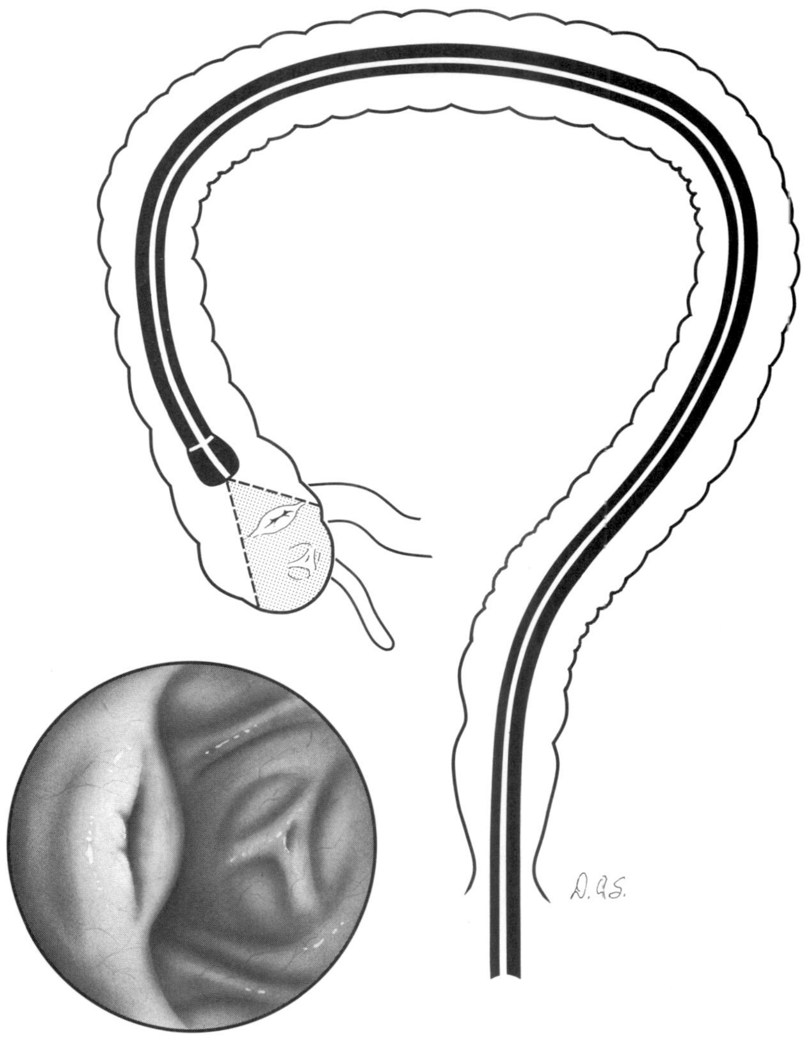

20

Colonoscopic Polypectomy

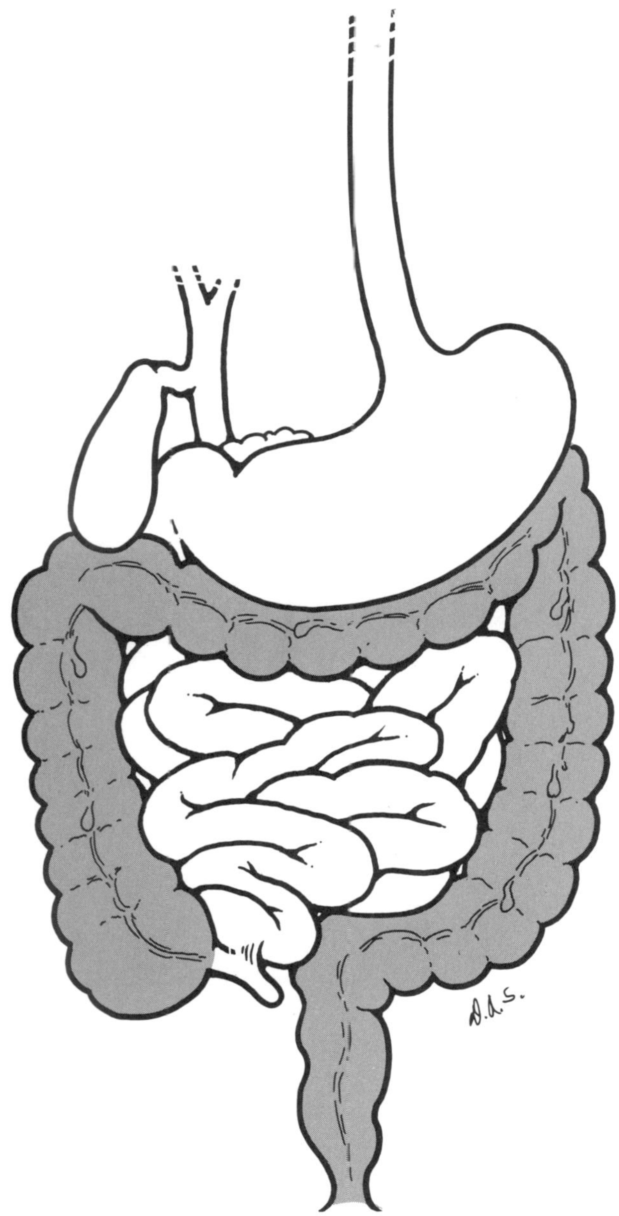

PLATE 20–1

Diagnostic colonoscopy has permitted the physician access to the entire mucosal surface of the colon, thus enhancing the evaluation and treatment of intestinal disease processes. The greatest therapeutic impact of colonoscopy has been the ability to remove neoplastic lesions. Polypoid mucosal lesions of the colon may be malignant, hyperplastic, or adenomatous. Submucosal lesions such as lipomas, carcinoid tumors, and leiomyomas may also occasionally be removed. Vigorous mechanical bowel preparation is required for polypectomy in order to clear the colonic lumen of fecal debris and to remove gases that may support combustion.

Small mucosal polyps may represent hyperplastic lesions or very small adenomas. Those that disappear with full inflation of the colon are likely to be hyperplastic and usually require no therapy, as they have no malignant potential. Small adenomas (2 to 3 mm) may be treated by "hot biopsy" techniques.

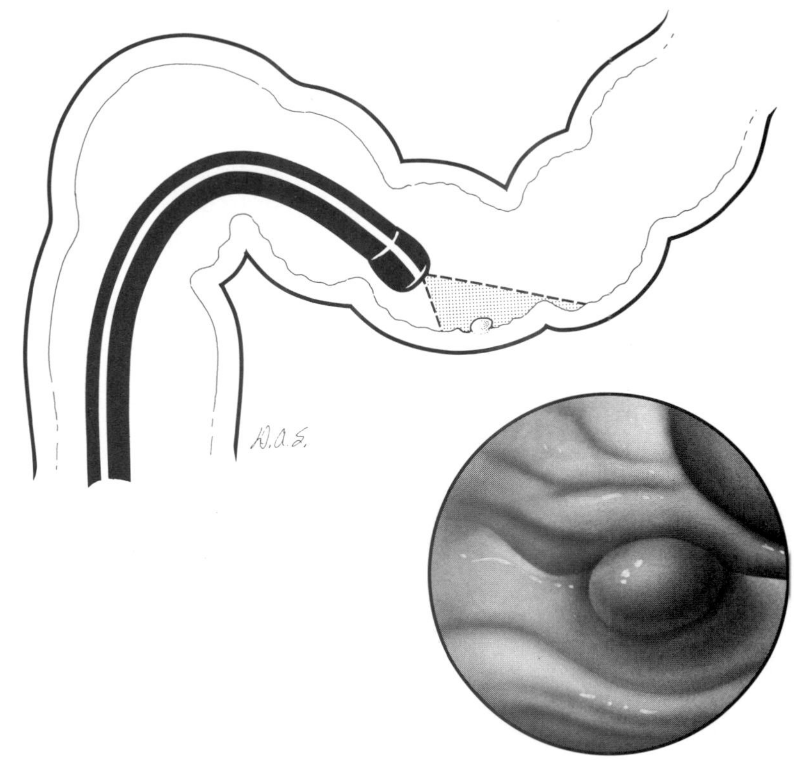

PLATE 20–2

The hot biopsy forceps has an insulated shaft. Its jaws are used to grasp the tip of the small lesion **(A).**

Traction is applied to the forceps to distract the polyp toward the center of the colonic lumen so that current is not applied to adjacent tissue **(B).** Coagulation current is applied in short bursts while tissue effects are evaluated. The aim is not to obliterate the polyp, but rather to create sufficient tissue damage to ensure that it will slough. A white cone of coagulated tissue appearing at the base of the polyp indicates that therapy is complete. Excessive application of current may lead to transmural injury and subsequent perforation.

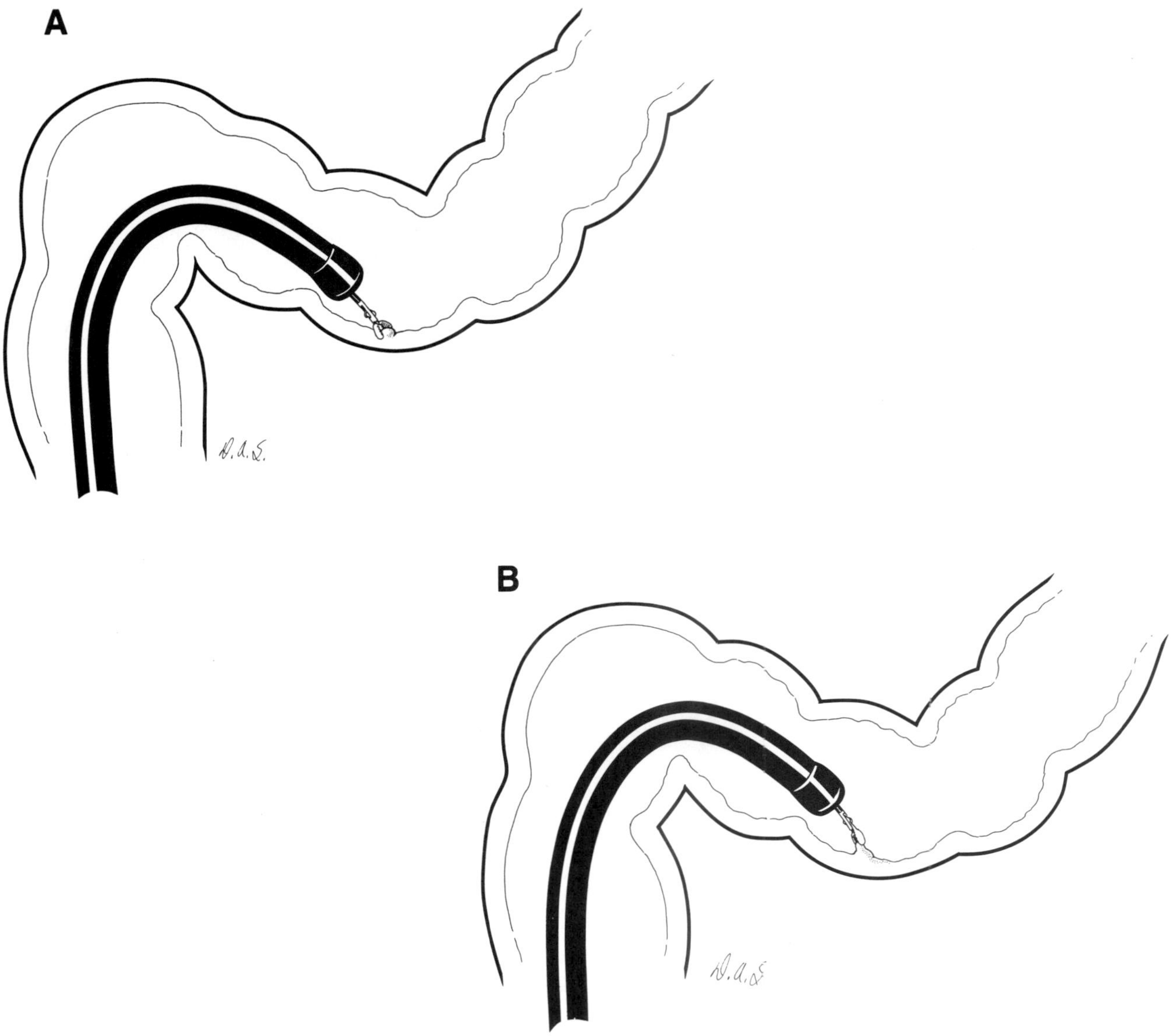
A
B

PLATE 20–3

After therapy is concluded a swollen coagulum will remain that is often larger than the original polyp. No attempt should be made to excise this, as it will slough in several days.

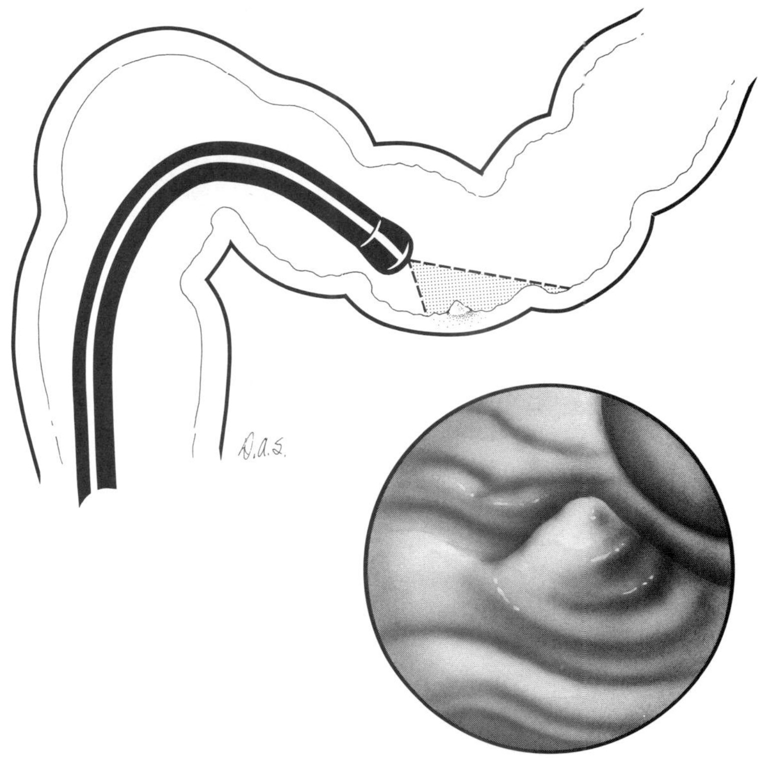

PLATE 20–4

Pedunculated polyps are common and may grow to large size. The malignant potential of these polyps increases with increasing size and the percentage of villous tissue present. Virtually all such polyps may be removed endoscopically. The head of the polyp is the neoplastic portion, while the stalk represents an elongation of the normal colonic mucosa. Transection is performed close to the junction of the stalk with the head of the polyp.

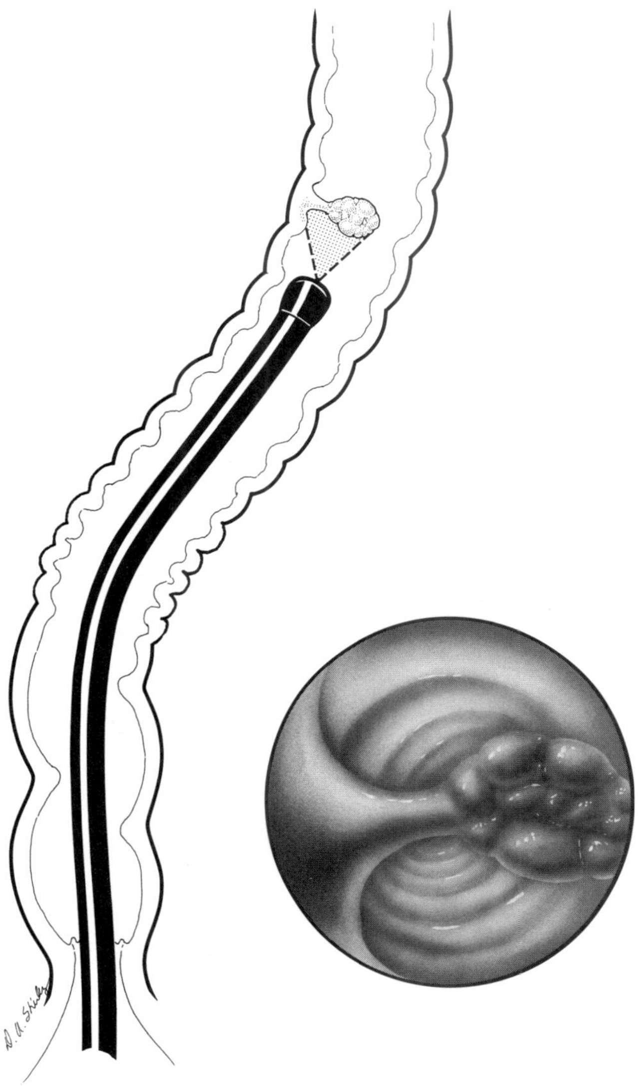

PLATE 20–5

The polypectomy snare is advanced into the lumen of the bowel and beyond the head of the polyp. It is here, in the proximal lumen, that the snare is opened **(A).** It is then pulled back until it comes to lie over the head of the polyp.

Once positioned over the head of the polyp, the snare is maneuvered so that the polyp's head is completely surrounded **(B).** If the polyp is too large to fit within the snare loop, piecemeal excision should be considered.

Once around the head of the polyp, the snare may be partially closed. The tip of the endoscope may be turned toward the bowel wall. A point should be selected for transection of the stalk, which is close to the junction of the polyp head and the stalk **(C).** The stalk is an extension of the colonic mucosa and there is no benefit in removing more of it than necessary to fully excise the neoplastic head of the polyp. Further, transecting the stalk too close to the bowel wall may lead to thermal injury of the colonic wall.

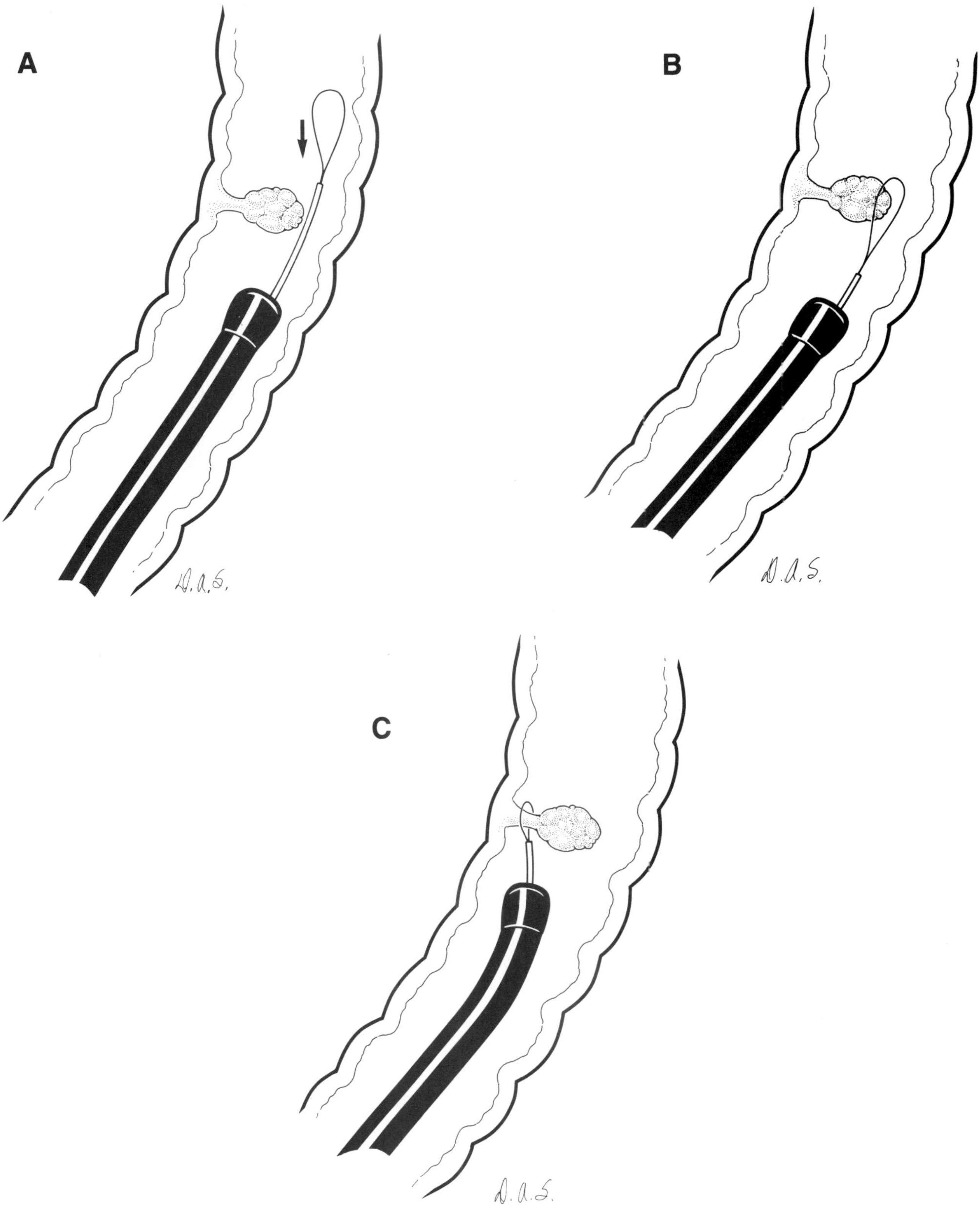
A
B
C
D.A.S.
D.A.S.
D.A.S.

To position the wire loop exactly at the desired site for transection, the plastic sheath of the snare should be placed against the proposed site. When the wire is tightened, the snare will close to the selected point **(D).**

Once the snare is secure at the site of proposed transection, intermittent short bursts of coagulation current are applied **(E).** This should produce a visible line of tissue desiccation at the snare wire.

The wire is progressively tightened until transection is complete **(F).** When the transection is complete, care should be taken to examine the remaining stalk and assure that hemostasis is complete. Should bleeding occur, injection with epinephrine solution (1:10,000) is effective in controlling hemorrhage. Repeat coagulation of the stalk is to be avoided.

The polyp may be removed by approaching it with the endoscope and applying suction **(G).** The instrument may then be slowly withdrawn with the polyp. Small polyps may be suctioned through the biopsy channel of the scope and into a trap. Large polyps may also be removed by regrasping the transected polyp with the snare and withdrawing the instrument with the polyp in tow.

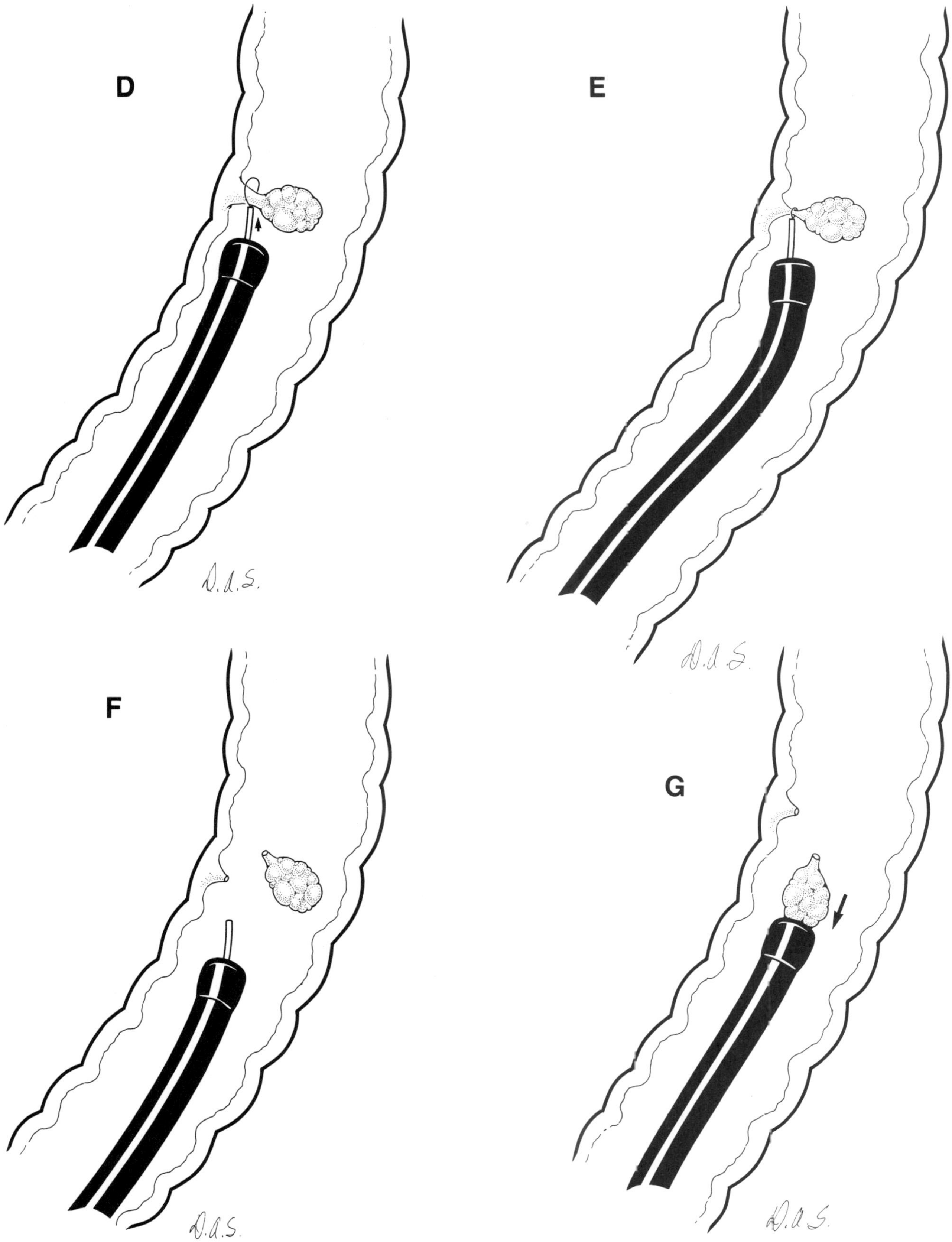
D
E
F
G
D.A.S.
D.A.S.
D.A.S.
D.A.S.

PLATE 20–6

Sessile polyps of the colon may also be excised with snare and cautery, but present a greater risk of colonic injury as they have no stalk. If large, they must be removed in a piecemeal fashion **(A).** This plate demonstrates the placement of the polypectomy snare around a portion of the polyp. Attempts to excise too much tissue at one time may produce thermal injury to the colonic wall.

A second portion of the polyp, along its side, is encircled with the snare in preparation for transection **(B).**

Multiple small transections may be required before tissue of appropriate size for final transection of the base remains. Such a tissue remnant is surrounded with the snare and efforts are made to avoid gathering excessive tissue in the colonic wall or adjacent to the polyp **(C).**

After complete excision of the polyp, no mucosa will remain at the polyp base. Thus, there will be an ulceration into the submucosa of the colonic wall. Continued coagulation at this site should be avoided as there is great potential for transmural injury. The endoscopist should strive to retrieve all of the excised fragments of polypoid tissue with suction **(D)** or snare and submit them for pathologic examination. While a superficially invasive malignancy in the tip of a pedunculated polyp may be adequately treated by polypectomy alone, any invasive malignancy in a sessile polyp suggests the need for colonic resection.

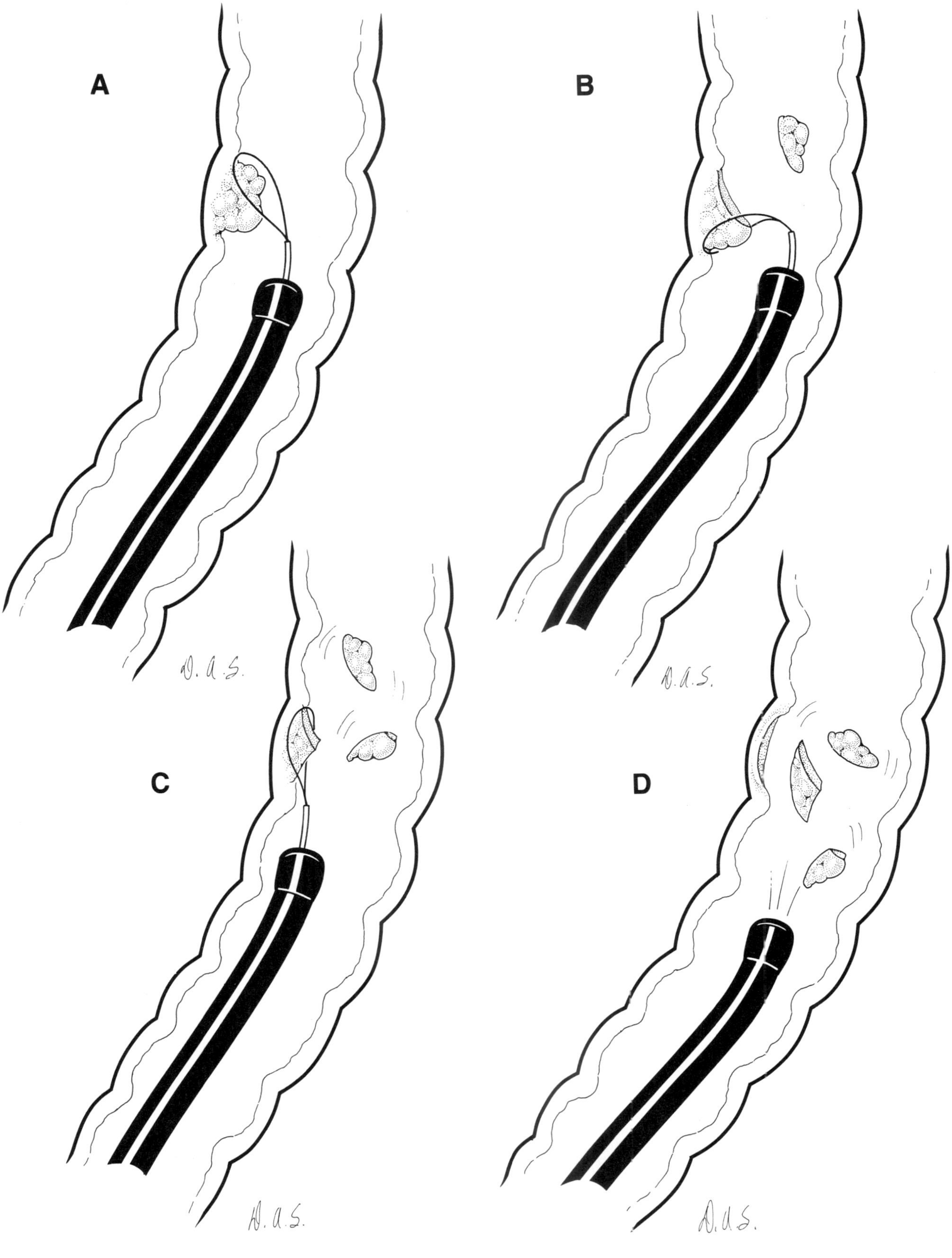
A
B
C
D

21

Colonic Decompression

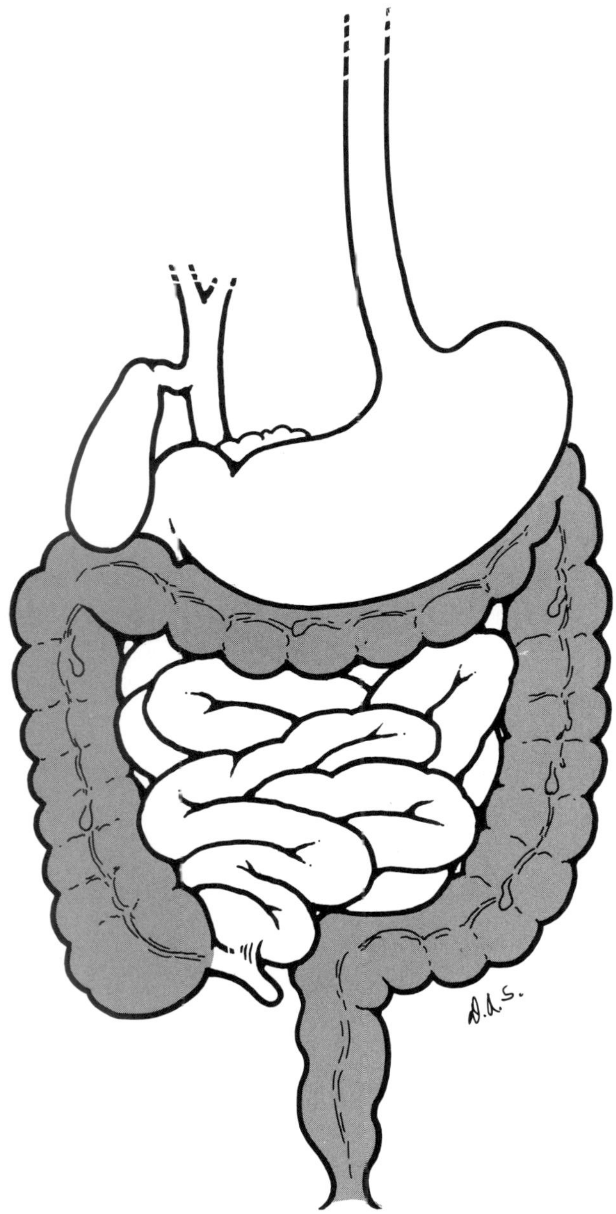

PLATE 21–1

Sigmoid colon volvulus is a commonly encountered problem. Traditionally, the volvulus has been decompressed by a combination of rigid sigmoidoscopy and placement of a decompressive tube. The colonoscope may be used to decompress a suspected volvulus. The instrument is introduced into the unprepared bowel and slowly advanced under direct vision. At the point of torsion, a twisting of the lumen may be observed. The scope may be gently advanced through this point, while keeping the center of the lumen in sight. The instrument should never be advanced against resistance, as perforation may occur.

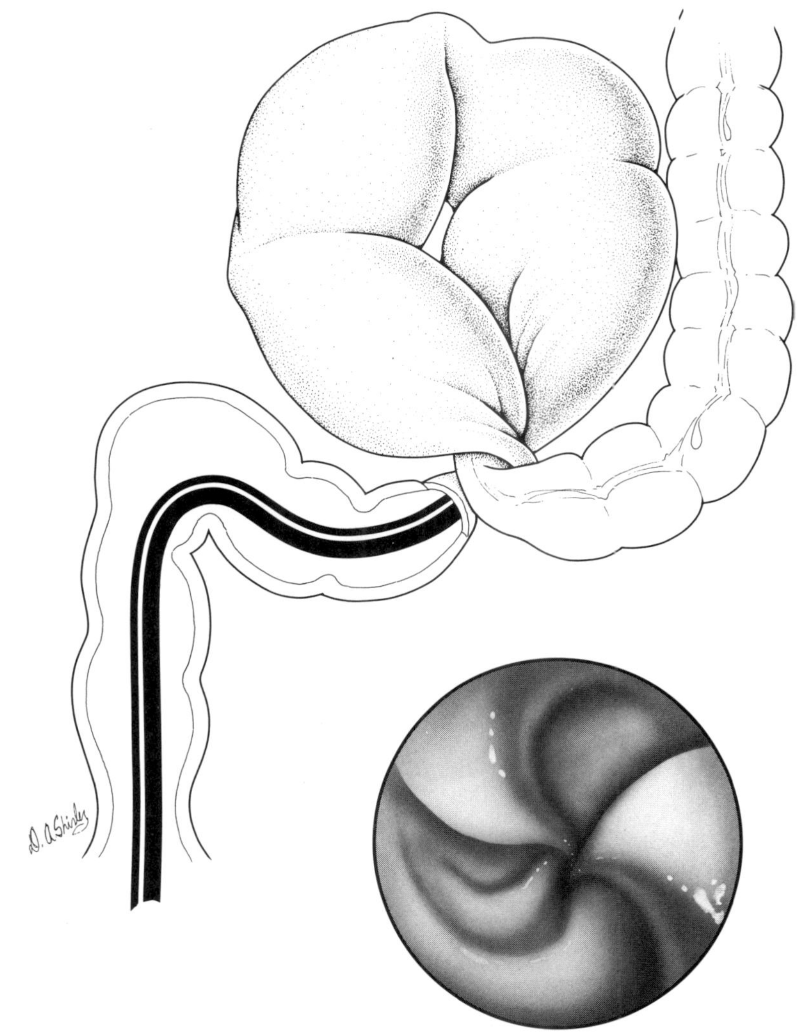

PLATE 21–2

Once the torsion is reversed, the proximal bowel is suctioned to produce decompression. The instrument may be removed and a biopsy forceps used to grasp a long suture tied to the tip of a large-bore rubber tube. The instrument may then be reintroduced into the descending colon. Traction is then applied to the suture in an effort to pull the tube into the colon alongside the endoscope **(A).**

When the rubber tube is in the desired position, the colonoscope is withdrawn. The tube will remain to continue colonic decompression **(B).**

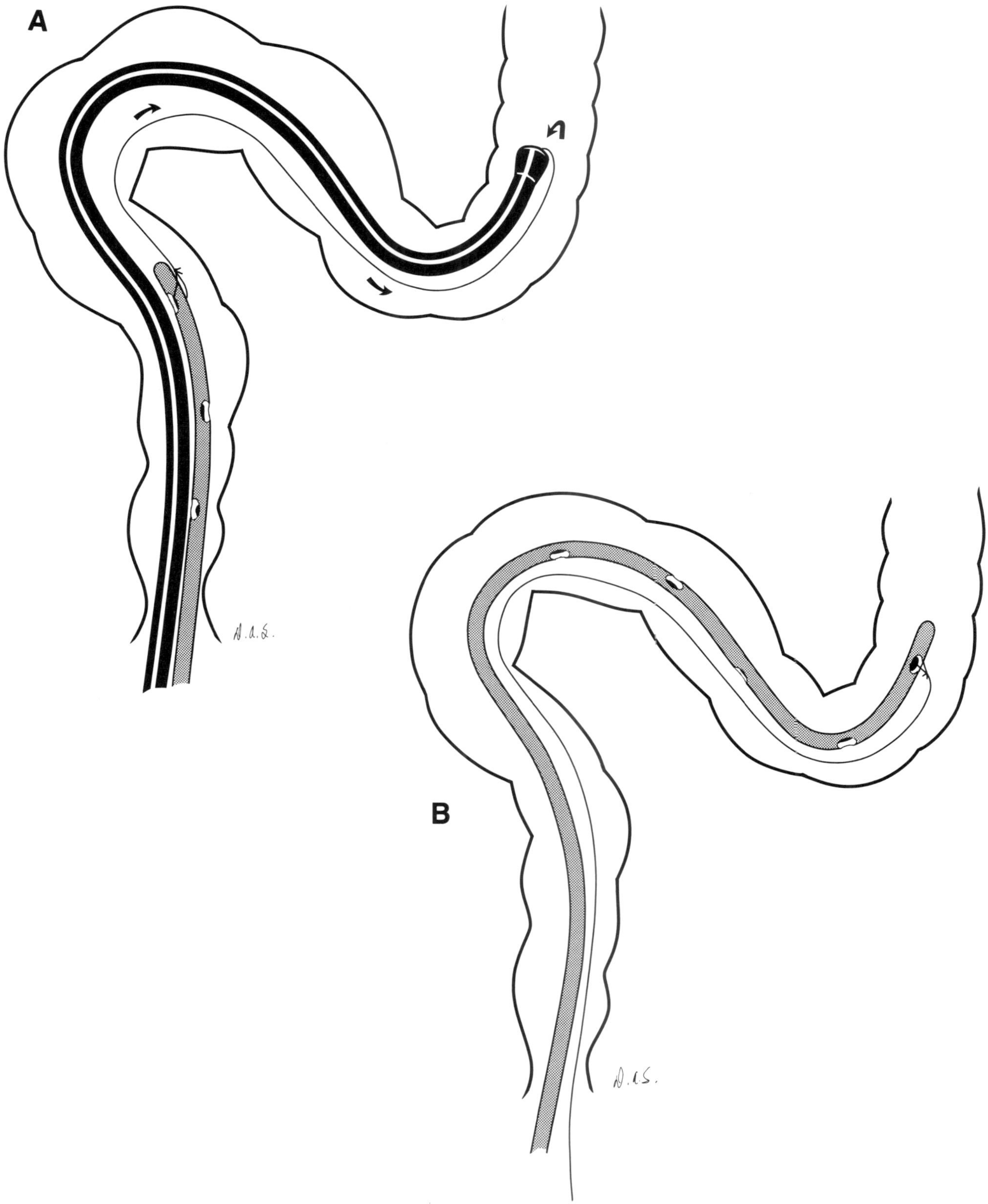
A
B

PLATE 21–3

Nonobstructive colonic dilation (Ogilvie's syndrome) is a frequent problem in critically ill patients. Colonoscopy may be performed in the unprepared bowel to decompress the colon. To maintain the decompression, a small-caliber, long rubber tube may be pulled through the colon alongside the colonoscope by tying a suture to the tip of the rubber tube and grasping it with a foreign body forceps passed through the biopsy channel of the instrument **(A).**

Once the tube is placed into the proximal colon, the colonoscope may be gently removed, leaving the tube behind for decompression **(B).** Frequent irrigation of the tube is important to maintain its patency.

A

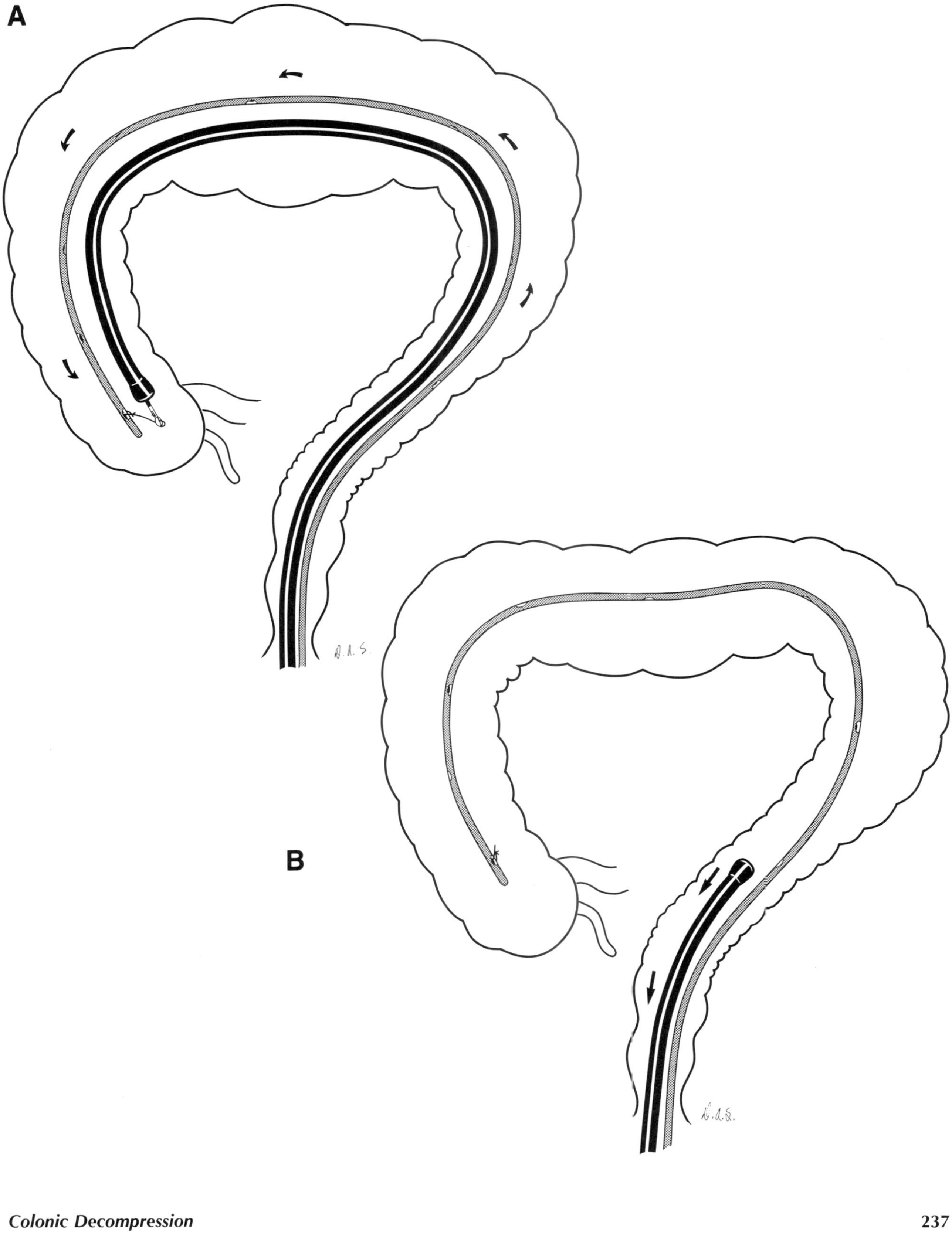

B

Index